LIFESTYLE SCULPTING

PRINCIPLES OF PERMANENT WEIGHT LOSS

ANNETTE RADVANSKY

National Academy of Sports Medicine Certified Personal Trainer,

Behavior Change Specialist, & Fitness Nutrition Specialist

DEDICATION

To Mike and Gianna,
my small family of big hearts.

TABLE OF CONTENTS

DISCLAIMER_____________________________________ix

ACKNOWLEDGEMENTS___________________________xi

INTRODUCTION_________________________________xiii

SECTION I: THE BASICS

BEFORE YOU BEGIN_______________________________1

1. MEET YOUR NEW CHEF________________________2

2. MY STORY______________________________________9

3. CHOCOLATE CAKE____________________________20

4. THE HEART OF YOUR FORMULA: SELF-DISCOVERY___25

5. THE PEMS SYSTEM_____________________________38

6. BRAINS & BRAWN______________________________43

7. SETTING GOALS_______________________________56

8. CHANGE YOUR FOCUS!_________________________61

9. THREE CONTINUUMS__________________________70

FROM STRESS TO PEACE_________________________71

FROM ABUSE TO NURTURE______________________74

FROM ENTITLEMENT TO SELF-HONESTY__________78

ARE YOU READY TO CHANGE YOUR VIEW?________89

10. THE SUBSTANCE IS THE SYMPTOM____________91

11. SUGAR: HOW SWEET IT ISN'T_________________101

12. DETERMINATION AND DEPENDENCY__________109

13. TRIGGERS___________________________________112

14. DUMP THE JUNK!____________________________120

15. FALSE BREAD VS. THE TRUTH________________124

16. WALK THE AISLES AND READ BETWEEN THE LINES_127

17. BRUSH YOUR TEETH!________________________134

18. NUTRITION LABEL COMPARISON_____________150

19. FOOD VACATIONS___________________________184

SECTION II: FORMULA BUSTERS

1: SPONTANEOUS EATING 194

2: NO PORTION CONTROL 197

3: FAT OR FICTION 201

4: OFFICE PARTY DISASTERS 203

5: RESTAURANT LUNCHES 206

6: BUSINESS TRIPS 208

7: NO EXIT STRATEGY 211

8: NO ACCOUNTABILITY 213

9: OBSESSED WITH WEIGHING 217

10: HIDDEN SUGAR 219

11: LIVING TO EAT 222

12: WANING MOTIVATION 224

13: RESISITANCE TO EXERCISE 236

14: INCONSISTENCY 244

15: CALORIE CONFUSION 249

16: OUR HUMAN CONDITION 256

17: DISCONTENTMENT 258

18: ALL OR NOTHING MENTALITY 262

19: CONFLICT IN RELATIONSHIPS 266

20: STOWAWAY FOOD 272

21: S-S-STRESS 274

22: NO WATER QUOTA 275

23: PEOPLE-PLEASING 277

24: CRASH DIETING 278

25: HOLIDAY HOLDOVERS 280

SECTION III: TOOLS FOR HEALTHY LIVING

1: WORK THE MOUTH, BUT NOT BY EATING 283

2: FIND A PURPOSE 284

3: CALCULATE YOUR SUGAR GRAMS 285

4: MOVE IT—DAILY 286

5: SWEAT____286

6: LEAVE THE KITCHEN____________________________________287

7: KNOW YOUR TRIGGERS__________________________________287

8: ELIMINATE MOST PROCESSED FOODS_______________________288

9: EAT MORE FOODS THAT RESEMBLE GOD'S CREATION_289

10: EAT MORE FREQUENTLY_________________________________289

11: ESTABLISH A WATER QUOTA_____________________________290

12: GET AS MUCH REST AS YOUR BODY NEEDS___________290

13: CUT BACK OR ELIMINATE ALCOHOL_____________________291

14: CUT BACK OR ELIMINATE FAST FOOD_________________292

15: MAKE A DECISION EACH DAY TO COMMIT TO YOUR PLAN, FOR TODAY ONLY   293

16: PLAY WITH YOUR PET___________________________________294

17: CUT OUT NON-FIBROUS CARBS AFTER 5 P.M._________294

18: PURCHASE MISCELLANEOUS MEASURING UTENSILS_295

19: PORTION YOUR FOOD IN ADVANCE____________________295

20: TAKE FOOD WITH YOU WHEREVER YOU GO________296

21: USE THE SAME SIZED BOWL/PLATE____________________297

22: H.A.L.T.____297

23: CHANGE YOUR MINDSET________________________________299

24: TAKE A COURSE OR HIRE A PROFESSIONAL_________300

25: BE CONSCIOUS OF FATS IN YOUR DIET______________301

26: PRACTICE SELF-EVALUATION____________________________302

27: MAKE THE BETTER BAD CHOICE_____________________302

28: EAT AT RESTAURANTS LESS FREQUENTLY___________303

29: LOOK AT THE MENU BEFORE YOU ARRIVE AT THE RESTAURANT____305

30: LOOK FORWARD TO SOMETHING EACH DAY_______306

31: SET GOALS BEFORE YOU RETIRE AT NIGHT __________ 306

32: CHECK YOUR HORMONE LEVELS __________ 307

33: PRAY & MEDITATE __________ 307

34: READ NUTRITION LABELS __________ 308

35: INCORPORATE JUICING IN YOUR REGIMEN __________ 309

36: SUBSTITUTE APPLESAUCE FOR OIL IN BAKED SWEET GOODS __________ 310

37: KNOW THAT YOU ARE IN CONTROL __________ 310

38: MAKE A CUP OF HOT TEA OR COFFEE __________ 311

39: PLAN YOUR FOOD "VACATIONS" __________ 311

40: CONTROL YOUR BLOOD SUGAR __________ 312

41: KEEP YOURSELF MOTIVATED __________ 312

42: POST QUOTES AROUND YOUR WORKSPACE __________ 313

43: APPLY THE 6-P RULE TO YOUR LIFE __________ 314

44: BELIEVE IN YOURSELF __________ 315

45: MAKE IT SIMPLE __________ 315

46: DON'T ROW IN THAT RIVER __________ 316

47: WRITE IT OUT, DON'T STUFF IT DOWN __________ 316

48: THEIR URGENCY IS NOT MY EMERGENCY __________ 317

49: GO ON A ROMANTIC DATE __________ 317

50: SIT OUTSIDE AND BREATHE IN NATURE __________ 318

CONCLUSION __________ 318

ABOUT THE AUTHOR __________ 320

BIBLIOGRAPHY __________ 321

ADDITIONAL READING __________ 325

DISCLAIMER

Although the author has made every effort to ensure the accuracy of the information in this book at time of publication, she does not assume and hereby disclaims any liability to any party for any loss, damage, or disruption caused by errors or omissions, whether such errors or omissions result from negligence, accident, or any other cause. This book is not intended as a substitute for the medical advice of physicians or other licensed practitioners. The reader should regularly consult a physician or licensed practitioner in matters relating to his/her health, particularly with respect to any symptoms that may require diagnosis or medical attention.

Information within tables is taken from actual nutrition labels and is for comparative purposes only. There may be additional data on the actual labels not reproduced in this book in order to maintain consistency and simplicity among all labels given. Due to copyright laws, no specific manufacturers have been mentioned or their labels displayed. If no value was given on the original nutrition label for a specific food item, then no value will be provided on the table. Product names, logos, and actual labels produced by the manufacturers have been removed to facilitate the education process. Actual numbers on labels the reader finds may be different from those presented here. Some names and identifying details have been changed to protect privacy. Any actual similarities are to be considered coincidental.

ACKNOWLEDGEMENTS

I would like to thank God first and foremost. Without my Good Lord and His grace, my life today—even my life itself—would not be possible. I hope I have glorified Him in this book, rather than seeking to glorify myself. I pray the spirit of service permeates these pages. May the results be His.

I would also like to thank my husband, Mike, for his unwavering support for me in all endeavors I have ever tried. There were many, and there are probably many more to come!

Gianna, my daughter and my inspiration, has catapulted me into another dimension of life and joy that I never thought possible. Her enthusiasm is infectious.

My editors, Joanne Hillman and Crystal Barnes, have taken my words and given them life. I believe God brought us together to help the readers understand their solution. This work would not be what it is without their devotion to this cause.

For these blessings, I am infinitely grateful.

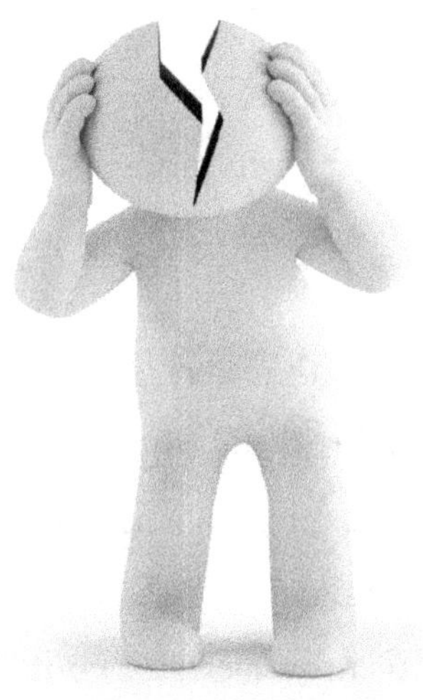

INTRODUCTION

"We can't solve problems by using the same kind of thinking we used when we created them." —Albert Einstein

How many of us have lost weight, only to gain it back and add even more pounds? We struggle and diet to reach that wonderful magic number on our scale. The truth is, only by permanently changing our lifestyles can we break this devastating cycle.

I too have experienced these 3 F's—*frustrating, fattening, failures.* Today, my life has been transformed. I am a happily married mother, a certified personal trainer, and am surrounded by wonderful friends. The formula that works for me and for my clients is the one I want to share with you.

If you actively work this program, I can promise you will begin to feel better. You will gain self-esteem and accomplish more worthy deeds in all parts of your life. And because you feel good about yourself, you will begin to treat yourself much better. You will want to take better care of yourself and maintain a healthy and nutritious diet. This will become an ever-upward progression:

Better health → more self-esteem → more worthy deeds → better health → more self-esteem → even more worthy deeds → etc., etc.

As a by-product to your efforts, you will find these unexpected blessings:

- Better relationships with others
- More mental, emotional, and physical energy
- A positive, rather than negative mindset
- More frequent smiles and laughter
- New direction and enthusiasm for your life

Many years ago, I was part of a social group. From time to time, I observed a portly member who never smiled. She seemed to be wearing a sign that said, "Leave me alone." One evening, she approached me and with brutal frankness said, "Annette, I have disliked you for a long time, and recently I realized why. Every time I saw you, I was reminded of what I wasn't doing for myself."

…Hmm. I began to think…

QUESTIONS

- Do you see yourself in this scenario?
- Do you know what actions you should take to feel better but consistently fail to do so? What do you think stops you?
- Do you have the desire to improve physically? Are you willing to make a move in that direction and do *something*, even if it is a small change?
- Does the wealth of information and misinformation available regarding food, nutrition, and dieting overwhelm you?

- Do you have a goal for your life? Or are you somewhere in between, on the fence, and indecisive about what you want?

- Are you willing to set specific goals and take action every day to achieve them?

- Are you willing to try the approach that worked for me?

SECTION I: THE BASICS

BEFORE YOU BEGIN

To find your lifestyle formula, you will first need to arm yourselves with facts about your personal physiology. The only way you can determine why you are overweight is to explore all possibilities. You must rule out the medical portion first. If you can afford the expense, get a full physical examination, with a panel of blood work if indicated by your physician.

If you do not have a general practitioner, now is the time to find one. Schedule an appointment and ask for laboratory tests to determine any medical reason for your excess weight. You may have to fast, so be prepared. After you receive your test results, take the needed steps to correct any abnormality.

When everything comes back normal, you are ready to begin.

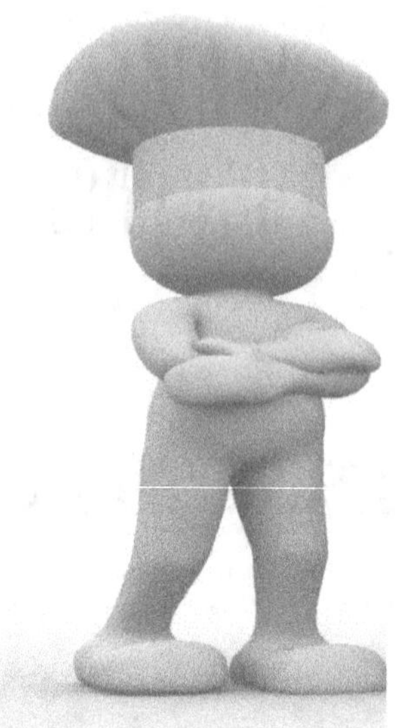

1. MEET YOUR NEW CHEF

"Great leaders are teachers not tyrants. They help their followers see and understand more. They inspire them to become more and motivate them to do more." —Michael Josephson

CHEF: Hi! I'm Annette, your new CHEF.

You: *Gasp! You're here to cook for me?*

CHEF: No, CHEF is an acronym for a **C**oach for your **H**ealth and **E**verything surrounding **F**ood.

You: *Oh, no. This is another diet book?!*

CHEF: Aren't you going to say, "Hi?" I thought you would be glad to talk to me! Hey, you might think this is just another book that prescribes a specific plan for you to follow so you can lose weight. But I have news for you. This is *not* a diet book, nor is it another fad. The information in this book will help you, not only to lose your excess weight, but it will also help you to maintain the weight loss for life.

You: *How can you say this book isn't a diet book, when all it talks about is losing weight?*

CHEF: I'm so glad you asked. I'm happy to tell you this book does not fall in those other categories. I offer no scientific hypothesis to diagnose your problem nor any diet plans or charts telling you what you should or should not eat. I do not list what you are to prepare for each meal, what you should weigh, or how much you should eat, (However, examples may be provided to facilitate a point here and there). In addition, you won't find the last pages filled with "mouth-watering recipes" to satisfy your appetite. You're not going to find a diet plan here, because that's not what this book is about. As you read and complete the practice assignments, you will design your own plan. You will find a resource filled with food for thought, nourishment for the soul, and appetizing alternatives for your life.

You: *But how is a book without recipes going to help me lose weight? You just told me what you aren't going to do. What are you going to do? I need a formula—a prescription. I need someone to tell me what to do, because I can't lose weight on my own. I can lose a few pounds, but I can't seem to keep them off. I need some structure and a plan!*

CHEF: You will find several themes throughout the book. First, I am going to convince you that self-examination is the answer to your struggle with food. Second, I am going to teach you how to get your own accurate nutritional information so you can make informed decisions, those right for you. Finally, I will teach you how to integrate your lifestyle and individuality with this information so you can develop your personal weight-loss formula that will work for you the rest of your life.

You: *I've got to admit, I'm intrigued. And come to think of it, I probably don't know as much about nutrition as I should, either.*

CHEF: You probably already know how to lose weight. You've done it before—perhaps many times. Are you still searching for a solution because you want to learn, not only how to lose weight, but also how to maintain the loss?

You: *Yes, that's right. I do want to know how to keep it off. So, let me get this straight. This plan has two parts: self-examination and nutritional information. I never tried working both of those at the same time. Maybe that's why I couldn't maintain the weight loss.*

CHEF: Losing weight and keeping it off are two different things, and also two similar things. While there is some overlap between the two, both have their unique challenges. Listen, if you want to lose weight and keep it off, you have to begin living as if you have already lost it. Learning how to do this may take some time. That's where this book comes in, and that's where I come in—your own personal CHEF: a Coach for your Health and Everything surrounding Food. That's me!

You: *Ooh-kay. Go on.*

CHEF: First, let's begin with a prerequisite. Do you remember those pesky things in school that you had to complete before going to the next course level? Well, there is one prerequisite for this book: HONESTY. I know it seems hokey, but here's your first homework assignment. Fill in the blanks below with your name, signature, and date.

PROMISE TO MYSELF

I, ____, will be as honest as I am capable of being for the duration of this book. This will begin a new way of life for me. I will obtain a notebook dedicated to the purpose of working the exercises presented in this study. I commit to answer all the questions asked of me and complete all the exercises given to me to the best of my ability. I may find that my level of honesty will grow deeper with continued study and exercises. I will allow myself to go back to certain areas and rework them for a greater understanding about myself if I choose to do so.

Signature____

Date____

You: *You are kind of goofy, but I like you. Okay, I did it. I signed that silly prerequisite, but I feel I'm a pretty honest person to begin with. I don't see why I needed to do that.*

CHEF: I like you, too! But I don't think you're goofy. Anyway, as you explore this book, you will find out just how honest you are with yourself. We'll explore your honesty by doing dozens of written drills, and through the process, you will learn to derive your own formula for healthy living.

You: *Okay, keep going. What's the idea with the notebook?*

CHEF: To complete all these written activities, you'll need enough paper for a lot of writing. I suggest you purchase a large spiral notebook for this purpose.

You: *Writing as a part of a diet? I've never been much of a writer. I'm not so sure about this.*

CHEF: That's all right. That's all I'll ask you to do—to start. You don't have to write well, because this is for your eyes only.

You: *Okay.*

CHEF: I want to emphasize that this plan is a call for self-exploration and introspection. I will ask you to self-examine as never before, because if you truly want the solution—the *real and permanent* solution to your individual struggle surrounding food—you will have to do some digging.

You: *It sounds too complex.*

CHEF: At first, it may seem so. Some answers will come from inside you. You have known these all along, but the homework assignments will crystallize—bring to the surface—some of your own wisdom. They will help you find a joyful new awareness.

You: *I'm going to need some help. I don't think I can do this by myself.*

CHEF: Few people can. Over time, you will obtain useful knowledge you may not have known. If you want further study, you may venture in to other nutrition-related resources. You may decide to hire a professional nutritionist or a counselor. Also, the internet has a wealth of information about exercise and body movement, or you may prefer to purchase a DVD, enroll in a class, or hire a personal trainer. Also, don't forget about supportive friends you can trust to keep you on track. Your customized formula will be comprised of many different techniques and sources of knowledge, all based upon the principles I'll show you.

You: *I'm a little uneasy. I've never done much 'introspection' before. I've never thought there was much to that. I just want to lose my excess pounds. Why do I have* *to do all this other stuff? I feel you're asking me to work doubly hard with things unrelated to my weight!*

CHEF: Let me ask you a question. How many times have you lost weight or gone on some kind of diet, only to regain the weight back later?

You: *More times than I care to admit.*

CHEF: Then can you understand why something more might be required for you to attain permanent weight loss? If this is your goal, you might need a different approach—not just another diet plan, but something *really* different.

You: *What do you mean?*

CHEF: The answer might be unrelated to the food, deeper than mere physical struggle. For many of us, our abuse of food is a by-product of something deeper inside of us.

For most of us, our abuse of food is a by-product of something deeper inside of us.

You: *Yuck. This sounds hard.*

CHEF: Yes, it is. But it works. Are you ready for the real solution?

You: *I don't know what else to do or where else to go. I don't really want to do this, but I feel backed up against a wall. I think you might be right. At least, I've never tried this approach. Like I said, I don't want to do anything uncomfortable, but I really want to lose weight and keep it off. I'm tired of this struggle!*

CHEF: It sounds like you might be ready to start.

You: *Yeah, I guess so, but let's hurry and get it over with!*

CHEF: No, it doesn't work that way.

You: *I was just joking. I'm ready. Let's go.*

CHEF: Awesome. To begin, I'll tell you my story and how I arrived at this place. I think you'll see we've both been in the same boat.

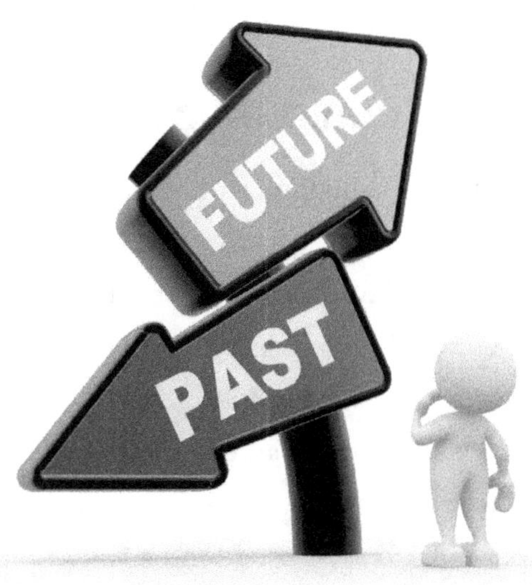

2. MY STORY

"But God demonstrates his own love for us in this: While we were still sinners, Christ died for us." —Romans 5:8

MY ISSUES

I suffered from low self-esteem, lacked any sense of identity, and always tried to be, look, or act like someone other than myself. I felt deep shame for who I perceived myself to be. However, a wise man once said, *"Things turn out best for those who make the best of the way things turn out."*[i] What I once thought was the worst time in my life turned out to be a gift. Through trial and error, I've had so much to learn about living a healthy lifestyle, I almost had to reinvent myself.

Although my story is not yours and you need not follow my same path, you may see similarities. But everyone is different and will travel a different route of self-discovery to find his or her own health and nutrition formula.

My hope is to help you have an easier journey than I did and improve your quality of life.

CHILDHOOD

I grew up in a home where drinking alcohol was the way of life. Every celebration included liquor, a lifestyle that ran generations deep on my mother's and father's sides. This environment set the framework for the person I was to become. I didn't know about the risks and pitfalls characteristic of children from such homes.

Because my parents (and their parents) didn't have healthy tools for living, they learned to cope with life by using alcohol. As a result, I followed the same pattern, except I used food as my coping mechanism.

My childhood was devoid of spiritual teachings, so I grew up an agnostic, even though I had no idea what the word meant. While I didn't have a rebellious spirit, the idea of God was foreign to me. So later in life, I resisted the concept.

As a teenager, I dabbled in binge-eating, crash dieting, recreational drugs, and alcohol—four addictive activities that would later come back to haunt me.

FRANCE

My world was shaken in 1982 at the age of nineteen. I was in my first year of college when I received an opportunity to live in Paris for one year as an *au pair* for relatives of mine. Excited, I began to prepare by adding French to my freshman curriculum at the university. At the end of the semester, I obtained my passport and my one-way ticket, packed my bags, and boarded a plane headed for Europe.

The next few months were jammed with new sights, sounds, smells, foods, cars, people, customs, and ways of life. People in Paris used public transportation much more than in America. They shopped for groceries in a market square with their own roller-carts, dumping vegetables and other items into the cart receptacle. People began their evenings much later and ended them in the wee hours of the morning. Late-night parties were held during the week. The workday started much later, and many had no lunch break. Everyone seemed to smoke cigarettes. The culmination of these small differences overwhelmed me.

Instead of embracing this new experience with zeal, I became isolated and filled with fear. Because I didn't speak the language, I was afraid to go out and explore. Although many Parisians spoke English fairly well, I stayed home alone while the children were at school. Since I didn't feel comfortable in the new culture, I didn't make any effort to assimilate. To pass the time, I ate.

I questioned everything. How do I dress? Should I speak to certain individuals? How do I address them? How do I fit in? I had been insecure and without a strong identity before, but in Paris, I had absolutely no sense of self. I was a lost soul, afraid to even speak for fear of revealing myself a foreigner.

I remember wearing blue jeans, a cropped top, and flip-flops one day, and being told these were inappropriate. "Ladies in Paris dress like ladies," I was told in a very condescending manner. My great uncle was the grandfather of the children I cared for. He lived in Houston, but he was visiting when I arrived. At home, he and I had a close relationship. But here in France, he criticized the way I dressed, and he accused me of saying things I didn't say. I was totally confused. His meanness will forever be a mystery to me, since he passed away long ago.

The way I had previously lived and related to others was challenged, and I had no one to turn to. This was before the cell phone, so I couldn't call someone without serious financial repercussions.

In addition, the parents of the children drank like fish. I had left one compulsive family for another. Already accustomed to this lifestyle, I didn't understand how susceptible I would be to such explosive dynamics.

Someone else might have reacted differently, but the way I

responded to all this change was to overeat. A different person might have embraced this new experience abroad with courage and enthusiasm. Instead, I shrank away in fear. I was out of my element, and I knew it.

Remember my telling you I had dabbled in various addictive behaviors that would come back to haunt me? Well, in Paris this happened. But since I was responsible for the children, I knew I couldn't use drugs or alcohol. A perfect storm was closing in on all of my bad habits at this point, and those habits concentrated themselves on one thing—binge eating.

In isolation, I ate constantly. And I ate and ate again. I would eat until I passed out. My weight exploded in a matter of months from a healthy 140 pounds on my 5'7" frame to almost 200 pounds. I almost died inside every time someone attempted to compliment me as "statuesque" and "Rubenesque."

I was out of control and filled with self-hatred. What kind of person was I, not to be able to manage something as innocuous as food? No matter what I tried, I couldn't stop eating. The more I tried to limit my food, the less constraint I had. I felt humiliated, yet my pride kept me from reaching out for help.

I finally reached rock bottom: physically, mentally, emotionally, and spiritually. No matter how hard an effort I made to stop overeating, I continued to get worse. My weight continued to creep up on the scale. I was desperate and fearful. I felt as if a monster lived inside of me, determined to kill me.

The thought of doing something drastic, such as taking my own life, never occurred to me. The human will to survive is an amazing thing. I just kept moving through life, one day at a time. Looking back, I think perhaps someone was praying for me. Someone was watching out for me, or Someone I wasn't aware of cared about me.

DISCOVERY

One day, I was walking along the bank of the Seine River and came upon Rue Quai D'Orsay, a street off the main river walk. A building with a sign, "The American Church in Paris," intrigued me, so I went inside.

When I opened the door, I found a small lobby displaying a variety of literature, all in English. With no one to greet me, I scanned the material on the table, not looking for anything in particular. My gaze fell on a newsletter. I picked it up and thumbed through the pages. I can still see the words in its margin, as if I were reading them now. *"Does the way you eat affect the way you live?"* An English-speaking support group met regularly for those who struggled with their weight.

The message spoke directly to my heart, and I wasted no time. There I found other lonely people. Their struggles were similar to mine, and they took me in immediately.

So relieved to have finally found a haven, I began pouring out my heart. My emotions were in a knot. I cried when I should have been laughing and laughed when I should have cried. This was the beginning of the end of my former life.

I didn't realize it at the time, but because of my desperation over my eating and my loneliness, I had stumbled upon a new way of life. This included talking about and dealing with my problems. I learned to face the emotions associated with my issues, rather than internalizing them.

Formerly, I had overeaten because I never knew I should talk to someone about the things that bothered me. I coped with life by abusing food. I had never felt safe speaking of my private thoughts, so I stuffed all my feelings down with food in an attempt to ignore them. However, they were visible to the world when the evidence showed up on my body as excess weight.

QUESTIONS

Please take some time right now to answer each of these questions in your journal.

- Are you using or abusing something in order to deal with life?
- Do you have healthy tools to cope with life, or are you using something unhealthy, such as excess food?
- Do you feel something isn't quite right in your life?
- Could your struggle with food be a symptom of the real problem? Is your excess weight a result of having this problem?

MY CHANGES

The first thing I changed was to connect with the people at the church—not just talking with them, but really communicating with them about my feelings. I developed a new level of self-honesty and openness with others.

The group assured confidentiality to all its members. This, I knew, was vital. Once before, I had lacked discretion in my choice of a confidante. I had been brutally honest about my eating problem to a "friend." The next time we were in a crowd of mixed company, she shared everything I had told her. Humiliated, I learned a hard lesson from this experience: know whom to confide in, and if in doubt about that person's trust, don't share. Today, I have friendships where we can talk about things to each other in total confidence.

QUESTIONS

- Do you have fair-weather friends, acquaintances, or social partners as your only friends?

- Do you have at least one person you could trust to tell intimate secrets about yourself?

MORE CHANGES

A second thing I changed was to become receptive to a Supreme Being. Before my experience in France, I never felt a need for a spiritual dimension in my life. My thought was, "Things are okay, so what good does a 'god' do?" When I became desperate as a result of my food problem, I became open to receiving direction and guidance from Someone more powerful than I.

IN A NUTSHELL

To summarize, I completely lacked healthy coping skills for living a successful life.

- I avoided situations I felt uncomfortable about, rather than addressing my feelings and growing from the experience.
- I had no relationship skills whatsoever. I avoided relationships when there was a conflict, rather than communicating with others.
- I never set any goals or had a plan for living.
- I never took risks to try new things or tried to stretch myself in any way.
- I needed an overhaul in all of these areas.

Connecting with other people and developing a concept of a Higher Intelligence resulted in the weight melting off my body. Once I began to live like this, I no longer needed the food to deal with life, because I had other, healthier tools to use. I began to take each feeling or situation as it came, look at it squarely, talk about it to someone, and deal with it. As a result, I lost eighty-four pounds from October 1983 to July 1984.

OOPS!

When my job in Paris ended, I returned to the United States, but I still lacked a sense of direction in my life. My dad was living alone, so I moved in with him. I probably should've found my own place, because I would have been spared the next few hellish years.

My weight was 116, and I was so thin, my menstrual cycle wouldn't come back for four years. I didn't realize I had become so controlling over my food, and soon became addicted to the adrenaline rush of under-eating and running.

I failed to get connected with anybody back home, even though I knew what isolation had done to me before. The knowledge of God that I acquired in Paris left me, and I soon started bingeing again.

I was terrified of gaining all the weight back and so determined not to get fat again, I forced myself to vomit after my binges. Little did I know this problem would result in even more devastation. Desperate and incredibly frustrated with myself, I continued this bulimia for nearly six years. My emotions reached another low, but this time, I was suicidal.

QUESTIONS

- Have you reached your emotional low point with food? If not, how much further down do you have to travel before you wake up?
- Are you ready for change?
- If so, write how you believe you are finally ready.

FREEDOM

I decided to attend a "Freedom in Christ" seminar[ii] by Neil Anderson, author of the popular book *The Bondage Breaker,*[iii] at my church in January 1993. The meetings were held Monday through Friday nights, all day

Saturday, and even Sunday. My weeknights were now filled, whereas I used to go home from work to binge and throw up my food. While attending, I slowly began to comprehend the teaching.

Toward the end of the seminar, the host invited those attendees who struggled with bondage of some type or anyone who needed prayer to come forward.

I popped out of my seat and almost ran to one of those ministers. I desperately wanted healing. Overwhelmed with my problem, I was willing to try anything to be free.

QUESTIONS

- Are you out of answers for yourself?
- Even if you have a little reservation about trying something new, are you at the point where you will try anything at all to get help?

These are difficult questions. Take as much time as you need.

"We can doubt without having to live a doubting way of life.
Doubt encourages rethinking.
Its purpose is more to sharpen the mind than to change it.
Doubt can be used to pose the question, get an answer, and push for a decision.
But doubt was never meant to be a permanent condition.
Doubt is one foot lifted, poised to step forward or backward.
There is no motion until the foot comes down."[iv]

FREEDOM (CONTINUED)

I followed two ministers, a man and a woman, who ushered me in to a small, private room. We began to pray for what seemed forever! They asked me questions about my past, and for every answer I gave them, there was a prayer. They asked me about my relationship with my dad, mom, sisters, uncles, and aunts. They asked me if I had a mentor or anyone I was close to. (I didn't have either.) They asked me about how I perceived school and home life. They asked me how I felt about myself and if I had any goals or aspirations. I can't tell you how long I prayed with these individuals, but I'll tell you this: I walked into that room a drowning, desperate person, and I walked out a free woman—and I *knew* I was free.

After leaving the room, I had the physical sensation of walking on a tightrope. I knew I was free, but I also knew I'd better be really careful to hold on to this freedom. And by God's grace, I have held on to it ever since. The day was January 30, 1993. Today, I have had over twenty-five years of freedom from bulimia and compulsive eating.

MY NEW LIFE

I purchased a membership at a gym and began weight training with a personal trainer. In 1994, I began training others. From 1995-2002, I competed in eleven fitness/figure competitions and earned money as a fitness model. My life has taken a 180-degree turn, and I have been transformed.

I married the man of my dreams in 1997 and continue to train clients. We have a beautiful daughter, born in 2005. Today I live a normal life and maintain a normal weight.

Sometimes people look at me and say things like, "I'll bet you can eat anything you want," or "You've probably never had a baby," or "Were you a cheerleader or something?" or "You've been skinny all your life, right?"

Now you know the truth!

Today I have freedom from the compulsion to put things in my body I really don't want to eat. The reason is this: I have continued to apply the principles in this book throughout my life.

These principles can become habits with you too and will ultimately help you to reach your weight-loss goals. I hope you will benefit from my pain and will learn from my mistakes.

So you see, this is my purpose for this book—to share my experience and help create an awareness to benefit you now and in the future.

You: *Wow. I don't know what to say. I haven't been that far down the line, and I'm still not convinced this approach is what I need. But I admire you for what you've been through.*

CHEF: I appreciate that, but like I said earlier, my hope is that I can help people like you to "nip this thing in the bud," so you can enjoy life as it is meant to be.

You: *Yeah, I definitely could relate to some things in your story—the frustration with myself, for example, and the feeling that I am getting close to my emotional low point with all of it. I feel like giving up sometimes and not even trying. But the frustrating thing is, I think I'm at my lowest point, or I think I am finally ready to control my food, and then I just forget about it and want to eat. I don't know what I need to do to become and stay motivated to control my eating. Can you help me?*

CHEF: I can try! I do want to say that I've not shared my story because I expect you to go through the things I did to get over my problem. I don't expect you to take a seminar, go to church, or get involved with a group of any type. Those decisions would strictly be yours. However, I have experienced your same frustrations. Consider this analogy I am about to share with you, and I think you'll understand the approach I'll take to help your situation.

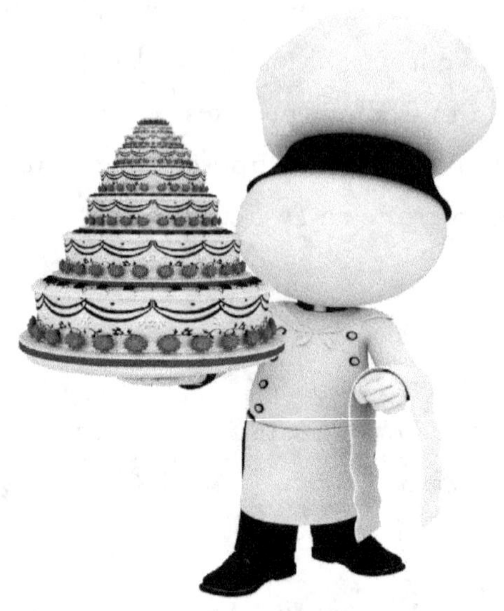

3. CHOCOLATE CAKE

"I praise you because I am fearfully and wonderfully made."
—Psalms 139:14

You: *You've gotta be kidding! Chocolate cake?*

CHEF: For every successful venture, there is a recipe, a strategy, or a formula the user follows. Think of this: how many recipes are there for chocolate cake? Thousands! But it's all called "chocolate cake," although the exact results will be different. Some of us might prefer German chocolate, Dutch chocolate, chocolate fudge, flourless chocolate, and so on.

You: *I have a great recipe that takes pudding in the mix.*

CHEF: You see, the choices are almost infinite. Even as you discover your preferred recipe for chocolate cake, you will design your own formula for weight management. Your program will be as unique as your own personality.

You: *That's a horrible analogy for a diet book: chocolate cake. It makes me want to have a slice.*

CHEF: I thought the "cake" analogy would be something you could relate to. In fact, I thought it pretty clever!

You: *I'm not really sure if I want to do this, but I do know that what I have done hasn't worked for me. Some of the things have caught my attention, things I never considered or tried, but I'm still undecided if I should trust you with my weight-loss goals.*

CHEF: I've told you the story of how I experienced a major weight loss and lifestyle change, but I'm not going to pretend I have it all together. I'm still seeking answers, the same as you are. Controlling my appetite is something I have to watch constantly, because I have a tendency to reach for food as a solution to my problems. Although I no longer overeat over situations or circumstances, the thought still lingers. Today, my struggle is more in my mind. And as you work through this book, I think you too will realize the problem of overeating begins in the mind.

The problem of overeating begins in the mind.

You: *Okay, I guess it won't hurt to try it. When I think about it, I realize that qualified individuals, like doctors and nutritionists, created all those diets I tried that didn't work.*

CHEF: My approach to food and lifestyle is different—not "one size fits all." Prefabricated/manufactured diet and exercise programs may work temporarily, but they don't work in the long run, because they aren't personalized. Many diet books prescribe a unique solution, supposedly for everyone. Perhaps it may work for one person, but likely not work for another.

You: *But they're based on science!*

CHEF: I appreciate scientific studies on controversial nutrition topics, because they help me gain knowledge and insight to make decisions for myself. Most of what you'll read in this book is based on scientific evidence, my own experience, or that of my clients. You are free to use what you need or to research for further information on a topic.

You: *I never tried the 'emotional' approach you are suggesting. It doesn't sound very practical. I want results!*

CHEF: This is a formula-finding book, not a diet book. It will become YOUR formula book as you personalize it with your notes, thoughts, goals, aspirations, and solutions. There are many introspective questions for you to answer, as well as suggestions you can implement. As you read each chapter and write in your journal, you will tailor your program to your own unique lifestyle and personality.

You: *I'm still afraid it won't work for me.*

CHEF: It will if you really want to change, honestly answer all the questions, and do the assigned drills to the best of your ability. If you implement these suggestions over an extended period, use the tools, and work on self-discovery, I promise you will most assuredly get results.

You: *Okay, I guess I'm willing.*

CHEF: I want you to lose the weight and maintain it for the rest of your life, and I'll ask you all sorts of questions. We are going to dig deep, so be prepared to get busy. This kind of work is rewarding and long-lasting. Please thoughtfully consider the questions I give you, because the more honest you are, the better results you'll get.

You: *Do I need to hire a personal trainer or nutritionist?*

CHEF: If you wish, you can employ qualified individuals to help you reach your goals, but keep their job description and your job description clear. You are going to do most of the work! And give this approach some time—at least three months, if not longer. Then, if you find this isn't working for you, simply put it down. But for now, let's start by taking a survey of your daily habits.

QUESTIONS

- Does your eating conflict with other members of your household, so you prefer to be alone to eat?
- Are you in a high-stress job in which you are frequently frustrated?
- Are you physically active, sedentary or somewhere in between? Do you want to change this?
- Do you enjoy your work, or is it just a way to get regular income and health benefits for you and your family?
- Are you experiencing personal stress, such as a move, divorce, death, separation, health issue or some other life-changing event?
- Do you have friends in whom you can confide?
- Do you have a spiritual dimension to your life, or do you feel this is not necessary to your happiness?
- How often do you eat out? When you do, is it hard for you to make good food choices?
- Are you a people-pleaser?

CHEF: These questions are for you to think about and write about. They are meant to stimulate your mind. As you honestly answer each question, you will make connections between your life, your general state of happiness, and your eating habits. You will begin to understand how your life affects how you eat.

You: *I think I could probably take these nine items and write quite a bit about each one of them. From what you say, I probably should. I'm really interested now. You're touching on stuff I never considered. I'm ready to learn.*

CHEF: Great! Let's go!

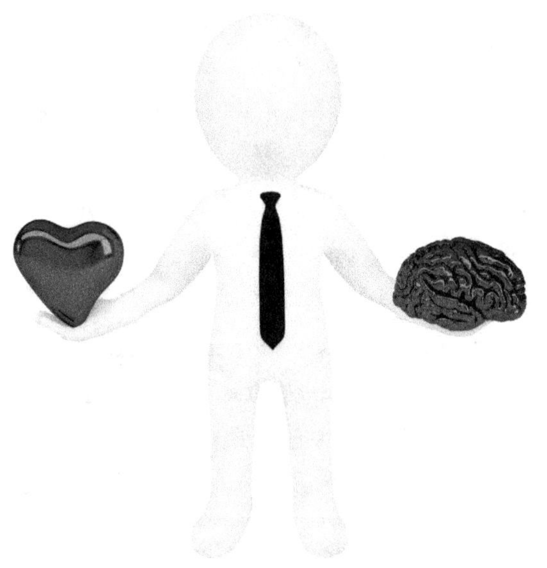

4. THE HEART OF YOUR FORMULA: SELF-DISCOVERY

"There is a principle which is a bar against all information, which is proof against all arguments and which cannot fail to keep a man in everlasting ignorance—that principle is contempt prior to investigation."
—Herbert Spencer

Spiritual hunger is every humans' longing to search for truth, to look outside of oneself for answers. Some answers are within us, but so many more come from the outside—through other people, education, our quiet times of meditation, and our source of Infinite Intelligence.

Many who seek balance in their lives have a daily quiet time to receive guidance. Escaping into a healthy, self-constructed cocoon is the way many of us find direction for our lives. To attain permanent weight loss, you will need to tap into this source of power.

Once I became aware of my spiritual bankruptcy, I began to change.

I had never previously sought anything or anyone for answers, inspiration, or guidance, but in France, when my eating spiraled out of control, I desperately needed help. I couldn't help myself, and I had nothing to draw upon at that time.

If I had developed a spiritual relationship earlier in my life, I might not have fallen so far. It was time I had a paradigm shift.

Cambridge Dictionaries Online defines "paradigm shift" as "a time when the usual and accepted way of doing or thinking about something changes completely." When we face a paradigm shift, we have several options:

- Do nothing
- Completely dive in
- Begin moving in a different direction.

Let's look at the options individually. Obviously, doing nothing will lead you nowhere. You know if you want real change, you must do some things differently.

The opposite extreme would be to dive in completely; i.e., to toss out your current eating plan and adopt an entirely new lifestyle. This risks burnout—doing too much too soon. You are likely to relapse into worse behavior if you are too zealous at the beginning.

This leaves the third option, to move in the direction of the shift. A different lifestyle takes time to develop. Our whole existence is like an unfinished sculpture. You must start where you are, patiently chip away at the block of marble, and slowly create the beautiful person you want to be.

THE HEART OF OUR PROBLEM

Perhaps you have no spiritual life. You may have never felt a need for one. Such a change may seem peripheral, unnecessary, and perhaps even a waste of time. Why pursue something you don't need? You've always managed to get things done without looking beyond yourself.

However, is it possible to have an emptiness and not be aware of it? Could someone live a certain way so long they become "comfortable," despite a deep, unmet need? Is it possible to become desensitized to or unaware of a need?

Take food, for example. Is it possible to eat a high-calorie meal, yet not consume any nutrition? Absolutely. Can we be full and yet desperately lack essential nutrients? This is more common than you might think. Is it possible for someone to be overweight and malnourished simultaneously? Unfortunately, it is.

The same analogy holds true regarding spiritual things—our souls, our inner beings. Spiritual hunger always parallels physical hunger. Even as our bodies hunger for food, so our souls crave peace. Could it be you have confused your need for spiritual connection with physical hunger?

I hear your questions: what exactly is spiritual hunger? Is there a way to identify it? Does everyone require the same amount? How can I develop this dimension in my life?

FEED YOUR SOUL

If you've been eating to satisfy your heart's craving, how can you meet that desire so your perceived physical hunger goes away?

I suggest you pursue truth that will feed your soul, even if you claim not to be hungry in that area. Why not try to break your fast with a daily taste of spiritual things?

Try this for a month and see what happens. Write your findings in your journal. You may be skeptical, but something is keeping you glued to this book. Curiosity is nudging you to look for answers.

I will also promise you an unexpected reward. If you begin this journey and stay with it for several weeks, you will establish a lifelong habit. You will nurture a relationship you never imagined between you and your innermost self.

Why don't you just try this way of life for a little while? If you find it doesn't work for you, that's fine. You can go back to your previous way of living. All I'm asking is that you try it for a short time. I believe by doing this you'll reap rewards you never expected.

I would like to offer a word of caution, though. If you begin this journey, you will not only initiate a habit, which takes several weeks to accomplish. You will also form this inner relationship. These will both take time to establish. What's more, you will need to maintain it afterwards.

A VOICE IN YOUR HEART

Listen for a voice in your heart of hearts. This is not a sound your ears will hear. Rather, you will sense an internal prompting you know is directing you for your good.

Allow yourselves as much time as necessary with this spiritual journey. If you remain faithful to this total program, including proper nutrition and spiritual nourishment, you'll find you have two separate and distinct appetites.

One appetite will be physical hunger, which you will learn how to satisfy with nutritious food your body needs. The other will be your heart's craving, which you will learn how to fulfill by nurturing your own individual spirituality.

At some point during this process of self-discovery, you might want to find a spiritual mentor or close friend of whom you can ask questions. Always seek the truth. Then you can slowly piece together what you have learned. Bring your questions, struggles, and challenges to your daily quiet time, expecting to receive insights. This practice, I promise, will change your life.

Where can you have quiet time in your house? Do you have a corner next to a window where you can stow inspirational books, your notebook, and pens? Designate a spot for these daily sessions. Gather your favorite materials. You will be more likely to continue if the area is personalized.

QUESTIONS

- Who are you, essentially?

- Why are you here? What is your purpose in life?

- If there were a God, what would He be like? What would you want Him to be like?

- Have you ever read a book or author that inspired you to think about these things? Keep these in your chosen spot.

CHECK YOUR SELF SUFFICIENCY AT THE DOOR

My agnostic environment as a child led to self-sufficiency as an adult. I was never interested in the dialogue of whether or not God existed. If He did, I didn't need Him. As a result, my self-reliance played a part in my downfall with food.

This may seem a contradiction. Shouldn't it be the other way around? Shouldn't *more* independence be the answer to any problem?

The answer lies in the fact humans were created to have a relationship with their Creator. If this fact is disrupted, and there is no connection with Him whatsoever, we are left adrift and defenseless.

BUT I HAVE TOO MUCH PRIDE TO BE HUMBLE!

Self-sufficiency leads to pride. Grandiosity leads one to think they can do it all by themselves. By contrast, a healthy sense of humility can be a source of great strength when we have a working relationship with our Creator. We gain a spiritual dimension in our lives. We change our priorities. We maintain a grateful spirit. We step down from our high horse and let Him have the reins of our life. We will enjoy weight loss as a by-product of our deeper change.

You: *Yuck! I hate that word, "humility." It sounds so weak.*

CHEF: I had a hard time with that word, too, but I hit such a hard and fast bottom with my food I was forced to look outside of myself. This made me humble. However, not everybody has to go through my process to be successful with weight loss. If you look at humility as an *advantage*, rather than a disadvantage (weak, as you said), I think you will see this frame of mind can be beneficial. This shift is part of the paradigm shift.

You: *Wow. I never thought of it that way.*

CHEF: If you are able to view your self-sufficiency as your biggest obstacle to long-term weight loss, then you'll see the benefit gained by humility. If you change your mindset, you will approach food in a whole new light, and the answers you seek will come to you with less of a struggle.

QUESTIONS

- If the way you currently live works so well in your life, then why are you still struggling with the food?
- What does self-sufficiency mean to you today, and how does it manifest itself in your life?
- Are you willing to let go of self-sufficiency?

You: *But wait a minute, CHEF. You are contradicting yourself. On one hand, you tell us that we have the formula inside of us. Now you are telling us that we need to give up self-sufficiency, gain humility, and look outside of ourselves for strength. This is confusing. Which is it?*

CHEF: It's both! As I mentioned earlier, you have probably already found you have many answers inside of you. You want to apply these answers with permanency. So, it may be necessary to look *outside* yourself for the strength to consistently implement your solution.

You: *Well, it's worth a try. It seems to have worked for you.*

CHEF: In addition, you may lack basic nutritional knowledge and need outside education.

DEVELOPING YOUR FORMULA

Your formula will consist of two dimensions. The first is physical, where you work to gather information about your individual lifestyle, portions to eat, and preferred food choices. We will do some of this here, but you may also want to seek outside help to set up a food plan that's right for you.

The second part is spiritual, where you connect with a higher mind—a loving spiritual Being outside yourself—for the strength to change your internal paradigm and achieve permanent weight loss.

The key to finding your formula is you.

The key to finding these two dimensions is you. *You* get to select what works for you in the food and exercise areas. *You* get to decide who to consult for information and how you will attain your goals. *You* get to choose how you will satisfy your spiritual hunger. All the choices are *yours!*

MELODRAMATIC?

"If your actions inspire others to dream more, learn more, do more, and become more, you are a leader." —John Quincy Adams

CHEF: Are you addicted to drama, or do you associate with someone who is like that?

You: *Now that's an interesting question. What do you mean "addicted" and "drama"?*

CHEF: Being addicted to excitement means to be in a habit of stirring up negative energy, conflict, and discord. Drama queens add fuel to that fire and then revel in it. These people love company. They pick fights and try to get anyone in their path to join in. If you aren't careful, they will involve you in their emotional turmoil before you know what is happening.

You: *Oh, I understand. I'll answer the second part of your question first. Yes, at work, I associate with several of those types. The first part of your question is a little harder for me, though. I think there are certain situations where I can overreact. I don't think I'm addicted to drama—that's a strong word—but I definitely have a tendency to get excited when something I feel passionate about is not going my way. I may pick fights with certain people too. It just depends on my mindset that day.*

CHEF: You might be drawn into habitual drama if you live or associate with such people. At some point, we have all experienced one or more of these situations.

If you don't tend to like turmoil, I want you to be more conscious of the people around you and learn to protect yourself from negative influences. Many dramatic people like to stir up negativity.

Are you often drawn into scenes at times, instead of standing aside as an objective observer? Journal each day, take action, and correct it. Becoming aware of what precedes your negative behavior is the first step toward a better life.

Finally, it may be hard to avoid certain people if they work for your company or live with you. One of my most useful tools is, "Their Urgency Is Not My Emergency!" In other words, it's okay to stay in our place of peace when someone right next to us is going berserk.

If you get an especially irksome drama queen who provokes you, it will be more challenging for you to stay calm, but it is still possible.

The more emotional stability I have in my life, the fewer theatrics I experience. Whereas the more spectacles I create in my life, the less tranquility I have. These are inversely correlated for me, so the more peace I have will result in a deeply satisfying and rewarding life. With this type of lifestyle, I am able to focus on things that are most important, like God, family, friends, and helping others.

You: *This sounds better and better.*

CHEF: Now, to bring this principle closer to home, how do you feel when you are on a roll and losing weight?

You: *Exhilarated!*

CHEF: That's great. You should be. Losing weight is exciting. Now, visualize yourself as having maintained that weight loss for five years. Are you still exhilarated?

You: *Probably not so much.*

CHEF: Do you see a contrast between new weight loss and steady maintenance?

You: *I do. I never thought of that before. But what's your point?*

CHEF: I used to fall in love with the process of losing weight, because it was so much fun. People noticed and approved. I enjoyed shopping and wearing clothes once again. I even developed more courage in trying new things, because I had a boost in self-confidence. However, when my weight was down for some time, I realized I still craved that positive feedback. I got bored with my eating routine. I regained the weight and started all over again. I was pretty good at losing weight, but I was lousy at maintaining it. This cycle repeated itself many times.

You: *Sigh. Yes, that's me too.*

CHEF: My point is to get you thinking about what long-term results look like, rather than the process. We all have experienced losing weight. This part is easy to visualize. Focus beyond the weight loss. What will your life be like as a weight-loss maintainer? What does this look like to you?

You: *I'm not sure. I've been so stuck on losing weight, as if that were my only goal.*

CHEF: And how about our daily eating habits? Most of our nourishment should be somewhat routine, with the exception of holidays and special events. Those times are appropriate for placing more emphasis on food and its preparation. However, the more drama I give to food on a daily basis—the emphasis, preparation, and time spent surrounding this act—the less healthful eating I am likely to do. Here, my expectations may exceed what the food is capable of satisfying.

You: *I guess you're right.*

CHEF: Conversely, if my goal is to increase structure around my eating habits, I free up space and energy to focus on other things. I will be free to be the person I am meant to be.

You: *I like that vision.*

CHEF: If you are adhering to your normal dietary routine eighty percent of the time and give yourself twenty percent of the time to have fun and plan your indulgences, parties, or events, then you should be able to maintain a healthy weight. It is when food becomes a priority one hundred percent of the time that we run into trouble.

You: *How do I begin?*

CHEF: Get a stable routine with your diet. "Boring" is okay when it comes to food, because you know you will be able to relax twenty percent of the time. You will take food vacations (I'll explain those later) when you invest more time and energy in your meals. You will enjoy and appreciate those special times even more.

You: *But what if my food doesn't taste good or I don't enjoy it? Aren't I more likely to relapse if I don't like what I'm eating?*

CHEF: Let's consider these questions individually. "It doesn't taste good" is an emotional response to rationalize bad behavior. I'm not saying eat something that will make you sick or that you don't enjoy, but it doesn't have to be exactly the way you like it every single time you eat. Always remember the primary purpose of food is to sustain life. This thought will help remove any emotional element. You will then be able to make more rational decisions about food and your choices. Just eat it, move on, and get busy with your life.

> ### The primary purpose of food is to sustain life.
> ### Just eat it, move on, and get busy.

You: *You're tough, CHEF.*

CHEF: The second issue is "I don't enjoy my food like that," and maybe even "if I don't enjoy my meals, I won't stick with the diet." I agree with this to a point, but the emphasis is most likely way out of proportion. Ask yourself if there is too much emotion involved in the process of eating. I'm not saying to have a bland, tasteless diet in order to lose weight. To the contrary! I want you to find tasty ways to improve your diets. Over time, you will learn how to replace unhealthy foods with healthier, more nutrient-dense substitutes. Greater nutrition satisfies the body more than processed or junky alternatives.

You: *I'm reluctant to say, I agree with you.*

CHEF: Armed with your honesty, you are the one who will decide what and how you eat. You select what to omit from your diet, some or all of the time. In addition, you are the one who will get the results from your actions. The choice is yours. Some sacrifices will obviously have to be made. Where will they come from? I think many of us have tried to have our cake and eat it too, for many years. I certainly did. It's time to put the "cake" down, think differently, and do the right thing with food. There's a way to find a new and better cake. You will see that you can enjoy your food and lose weight at the same time. Now, *that* is truly a gift.

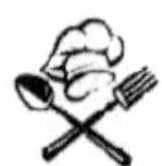

HOMEWORK

1. Do you feel you have any kind of emotional attachment to food? Clearly identify these emotional attachments. Write them down in your journal. Begin to make a sincere attempt to detach them completely from your eating behavior.

2. Take five minutes right now to visualize yourself at your goal weight. Record the details. Recall them into your memory every day. You can have this be a part of your daily quiet time.

SUMMARY

Eating clean and healthy during the week and then taking a small break over the weekend is a way of life, not a yo-yo diet. We want to behave in a manner we will be able to stay consistent with for the rest of our lives, so it must be comfortable.

Remember you'll probably make a few small changes to your diet at first. As you hold on to these few changes, they will be cumulative to the ones you add in the future. We are creating a sculpture here, chiseling slowly away at destructive habits and finding the beautiful person inside.

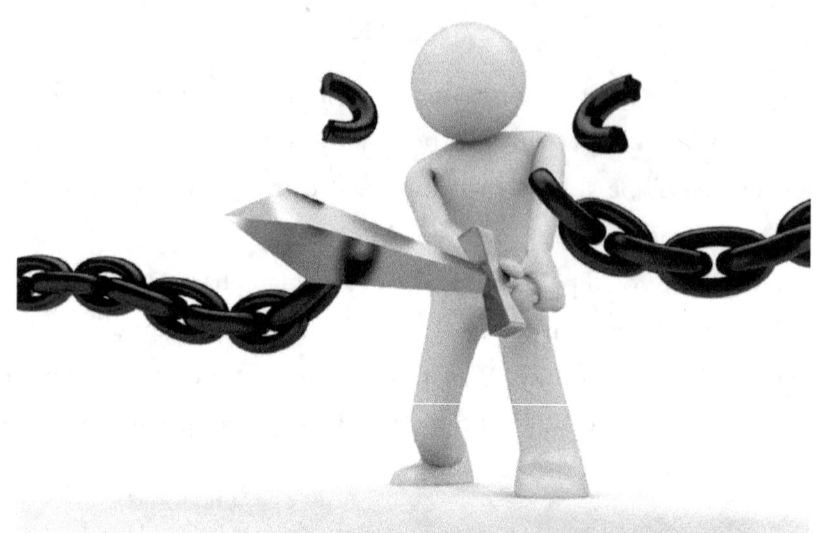

5. THE PEMS SYSTEM

"We are not human beings having a spiritual experience. We are spiritual beings having a human experience." —Teilhard Chardin

CHEF: To sum up all of my philosophy for you, I want to share something I learned from a friend of mine, years ago. It's the PEMS system. An acronym that stands for

Physical,

Emotional,

Mental, and

Spiritual.

The PEMS system is simply balancing all four legs of our "table" of life, so it remains strong and steady. It means feeding each one of these dimensions in our lives on a regular basis. When we do this, we attain a balanced and happy existence.

You: *This is truly a different way of looking at and living life. The analogy of the four legs makes it clear how I need to help myself. (1) My body is my responsibility,* *and I can choose wisely, through diet and activity, to see I maintain good health. (2) I need to pay attention to my emotions, because they can indicate if I'm staying peaceful. If I'm not calm, I need to change something. (3) Mentally, I need to stimulate my mind and always be learning something new. This keeps life interesting. (4) And finally, the spiritual part. This is where I think I have the most work. I'm beginning to understand I have a responsibility here too, to develop and maintain a relationship with God each day.*

I realize no one else can do it for me. I understand I haven't been taking responsibility for the things only I can take care of. I think this system might actually work for me. I feel a little overwhelmed, but I can't believe I'm also feeling a glimmer of hope! I apologize for being skeptical. This really makes sense.

CHEF: I understand your skepticism, and there's no need to apologize. Here's an example of what each leg, or element, might look like:

- **Physical:** We make good nutritional food choices and eat healthy portions. We exercise regularly.
- **Emotional:** We have someone we can always confide in. We nurture relationships with our loved ones, friends, and family.
- **Mental:** We engage in activities that stimulate our minds. We regularly challenge ourselves to do better at our work.
- **Spiritual:** We have daily quiet time. We nurture our relationship with our God.

Since we are made with all four of these elements, doesn't it make sense we should regularly nurture each one?

You: *It sure does, and I can add to those right now. How about making sure I get enough rest?*

CHEF: Excellent! Why didn't I think of that? What else would you add?

You: *Let's see… I could add a daily 5-minute journaling session as an emotional release. I could commit to leisure reading an hour a day for my mind. I could commit* *to meditation several times a week as a spiritual activity and to reduce stress.*

CHEF: Those are great examples.

You: *I see how the legs of the stool can help balance my life and make the other legs more enjoyable. For example, I see how meditation (a spiritual practice) can actually help me lose weight (a physical endeavor), simply because I'm not eating as a result of stress. I can also see how exercising can help me keep positive about life.*

HOMEWORK

Make a chart with all four of these elements and jot down at least two for each one that would apply to your life today. Take note of the areas you want to improve and how you could change them. Your chart might look something like this:

PHYSICAL	EMOTIONAL	MENTAL	SPIRITUAL
Find and visit a nutritionist to get on a healthy eating plan.	Set a weekly date with my spouse.	Read one hour each day.	Journal five minutes each day about my feelings.
Exercise five times a week, thirty minutes a day, alternating days of yoga and walking.	Call my sister once a week to chat	Join a writing club.	Meditate twenty minutes, three times per week. Find and download meditation music.

ARE YOU A COMPULSIVE OVEREATER?

Food addiction can be as destructive as that of alcohol or narcotics. The behavior patterns are similar, but with different substances. Support groups may help for severe cases.

The following questions are used by permission from Overeaters Anonymous (www.oa.org).[v] These may help you determine if you have an eating problem. Assess yourself honestly.

- Do I eat when I'm not hungry, or not eat when my body needs nourishment?

- Do I go on eating binges for no apparent reason, sometimes eating until I'm stuffed or even feel sick?

- Do I have feelings of guilt, shame, or embarrassment about my weight or the way I eat?

- Do I eat sensibly in front of others and then make up for it when I am alone?

- Is my eating affecting my health or the way I live my life?

- When my emotions are intense—whether positive or negative—do I find myself reaching for food?

- Do my eating behaviors make me or others unhappy?

- Have I ever used laxatives, vomiting, diuretics, excessive exercise, diet pills, shots, or other medical interventions (including surgery) to try to control my weight?

- Do I fast or severely restrict my food intake to control my weight?

- Do I fantasize about how much better life would be if I were a different size or weight?

- Do I need to chew or have something in my mouth all the time: food, gum, mints, candies, or beverages?

- Have I ever eaten raw food that should have been cooked? Have I eaten unheated, burned, frozen, or spoiled food? Have I been so eager that I eat directly from containers on the way home from the grocery store? Have I removed food from garbage and eaten it?

- Are there certain foods I can't stop eating after having the first bite?

- Have I lost weight with a diet or "period of control" only to be followed by bouts of uncontrolled eating and/or weight gain?

- Do I spend too much time thinking about food, arguing with myself about whether or what to eat, planning the next diet or exercise cure, or counting calories?

Are your answers "yes" to several of these questions? If so, it is possible that you have, or are well on your way to having, an overeating or compulsive overeating problem. If most of your responses were "yes," you may need to see a professional trained in eating disorders.

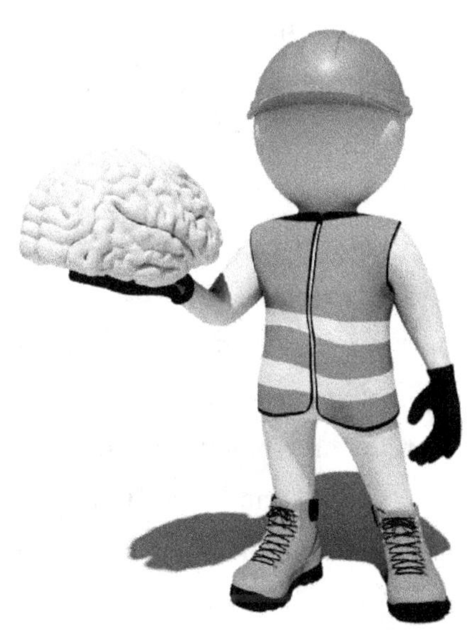

6. BRAINS & BRAWN

"The strongest principle of life and blessings lies in our choice. Our life is the sum result of all the choices we make, both consciously and unconsciously. If we can control the process of choosing, we can take control of all aspects of our life. We can find the freedom that comes from being in charge of our life. So start with what is right rather than what is acceptable. If you don't make a decision, then time will make it for you, and time will always side against you!" —Billy Graham

The focus of Brains & Brawn is self-analysis. Be prepared to write a lot. You will be encouraged to reveal, recognize, and accept—or change—certain things about yourself. This is the "brains." Your awareness will increase from the depth of your honesty. You will be rewarded for your persistence in working through the questions and written drills. This is the "brawn."

Do as much writing as you can. You will benefit from the process in several ways. You will find emotional relief for burdens you have carried. Suddenly, they will be lifted as you face them square on.

Spiritually, you will form a team with God. He is on your side and wants you to win. Physically, you will find more strength to care for your body. You will be more likely to succeed with weight loss and ultimately a lifetime of weight maintenance. The harder you work your mind in Brains & Brawn, the easier your work will be to change your food.

Consequently, less effort may result in no lost weight. Brains & Brawn is a section that needs the most time to develop. You may want to begin by simply reading it all the way through. The second time you read, take notes in the margins and highlight those areas that resonate with you. By the third reading, you will be ready to work the questions and drills. I cannot emphasize the importance of putting in the utmost effort and time into this section of the book.

THE DIURNAL JOURNAL

It's funny how journaling works. Once your pen touches the paper, words begin to flow automatically.

If you haven't already done so, get an 8½" x 11" lined notebook or pad to journal your thoughts every day. You will record anything that comes to your mind at least one time per day.

If you have never kept a journal before, it's really not a big deal. The most difficult part might be making it a daily habit. So whether it is easy or hard for you to write, do it anyway. You will find that journaling helps your mind become more efficient in all that you do. You will record private, personal items in there, so keep it in a safe place. This is an exciting time for you, the beginning of a rewarding process!

Your notebook will contain unstructured content from your random journaling. It will also include structured material from the questions and homework assignments.

PUT THE FOOD DOWN!

Through the work you do here, you may discover ways you use the food as a crutch. Some common themes are to cover your feelings, isolate, or react inappropriately to something stressful. It's time to let go of our unhealthy attachments to food.

Some of us have established bad habits over many years. Breaking these will take practice, but will become easier with time. Some suggestions I give you may not appeal to you. You might want to give others a trial run. Take what will work for you and put the others aside for later. You are here to explore.

You will read, write, and personalize your own process for healthy living. I will also share with you all the information that has facilitated my own and my clients' success. This will be an unbeatable combination for your new lifestyle, and your lifestyle becomes who you are.

HOMEWORK

- **Identify circumstances you want to change.** In your journal, list five circumstances in your life you would like to see changed, removed, or added to your life. Don't think about cost, time involvement, or any other constraints. Simply list them, and put today's date on the paper. To measure your progress toward a certain goal, it helps to see how far you have come. When you date your list, you will be able to reflect on your progress later on. Failure to develop long-term relationships, difficulty to retain customers, and poor time management skills are several examples.

- **Identify habits you do not like.** List two habits that prevent you from being the person you want to be. Shyness, overspending, and tardiness are several examples.

- **Identify healthy and unhealthy tools you use.** Whether you know it or not, you have tools for living. Everyone does. Behaviors you acquired during childhood may have served you well then, but may need to be upgraded, amended, or discarded. You may have tools to cope with current life situations. Become aware of these tools, and evaluate them to see if they need to be overhauled. The first step in making constructive change with anything is awareness. To know where you are at this moment gives you a starting point. It will also give you an idea of how far you need to go to reach your goal.

- **List one healthy and unhealthy tool you use.** An example of a healthy tool is to talk to a friend to relieve stress. An unhealthy tool might be to suppress anger toward someone with whom you need to communicate.

> ## The first step in making constructive change is awareness.

Refer back to the lists that you made above. Taking one item at a time, write one 8½" x 11" page of your thoughts behind each entry. Record where you believe this circumstance or habit originated. Why do you believe you started using it? Did you learn this behavior from a parent, relative, or friend? Did it occur as a knee-jerk reaction (an automatic response) to something that previously happened in your life?

Consider your list again. Can you identify where your tools came from? Do you use food (or something else, like alcohol, spending money, gambling, or depression) as a tool to cope? Are you trying to escape from uncomfortable situations? Do you need healthier ways to relax and unwind?

Once you realize how these behaviors originated, you will have a better understanding of yourself and how you react to life in different ways. Furthermore, you will be better able to make choices that will be more closely aligned with what you want today.

Here's an example of someone working through this process:

1. Circumstance I want to change: I don't like my body, and I would like to have more confidence in the way I look.

My thoughts: I've never liked my body. I'm not comfortable in my body. I don't see any beauty in it. Mom didn't like her body—seemed to be ashamed of it. I thought she had a pretty body, but she always seemed to be hiding so I couldn't see it. I think I'm ashamed of my body, and I don't know why. I guess I'm just like my mom. I know I overeat and feel I abuse myself with the food. I know I could probably feel better about myself if I lost weight and exercised more. I just can't seem to get myself out of this fix. I feel so alone. Maybe I need a friend—a really close friend I can confide in, and we can lose weight together. I want to be me and not my mom. How can I break this unhealthy bond?

My tool is overeating because I don't have courage to let people see me for who I am. The extra fat acts like a barrier to keep people away.

2. Habit I do not like: I only like to eat alone. I don't like to dine around people, because I can't consume all I want.

My thoughts: I have been doing this behavior all my life. My parents criticized me for my weight when I was seven and put me on diets. I started sneaking my food whenever I could. I felt I was getting away with something and eating made me feel free. When I ate, I felt I was in control. No one could touch me. When I got fat, no one wanted to be close to me because I looked different. I continued to isolate myself from others, and I continue to do that today. I feel like a social outcast because of my size. I feel there is no hope for me, so I just keep doing this behavior. I want to change and to be thin. Maybe I'm too isolated. Maybe I need to get out more and do more things with other people.

My tool is that I'm still angry with my parents. I stay fat, and I stay mad. Maybe if I worked to lose the weight, I would lose the anger toward my parents, too. Or, vice-versa.

3. Healthy and unhealthy tools: I am open-minded and willing to change. When I've been hurt, I withdraw.

My thoughts: Being open-minded is one of my strengths. Sometimes it backfires because I can be too trusting. I want to trust people because I want friends. But not all people can be trusted. I need to develop discernment. How can I do this?

My healthy tool is my ability to listen to others. I need to become a better judge of character so I can protect myself from mean people.

Withdrawing when I've been hurt is unhealthy. I use this tool because I am afraid to confront the person. My dad would yell at me if I asked him questions about anything. I think I'm still afraid of my dad yelling at me. I'm afraid of not being liked.

SUMMARY

To summarize, you are working on increasing your self-awareness. For some of you, this is going to be a lot of work. You will have to do some digging to get there, and it may take a little time. It may not be easy to look at, either. But be assured—the reward is well worth the effort. You will gain a greater sense of self-awareness and a newfound freedom. You will have determination to get where you want to go.

I know you are eager to get change in your life, but let's just focus on this part for now. Once you are done, you'll be armed with new knowledge. You will become more content, because you will gain a better understanding of yourself. Your self-respect will increase. You will be eager to change what you are currently doing with your food. These changes will become easier because of this advance work.

MAKE YOUR BED!

What you do today has a ripple effect on your future. You know the expression, "You've made your bed, now lie in it." This statement is all about the consequences of the choices you and I have made throughout our lives. Let's start facing the reality of our situation and look at the bed we are making for ourselves in five, ten, or twenty years from now.

I have trouble feeling sorry for someone who has spent years abusing their body and then wakes up one day with a health-related problem as a direct result of a bad diet and no activity. Do they wonder why? Information was out there. Self-honesty was available to them. The bad news is their lifestyle finally caught up to them, and they suddenly have a serious health problem on their hands.

Many problems related to a bad diet and lifestyle are reversible.

The good news is many of these problems related to a bad diet and lifestyle are reversible. Diabetes (type II), high blood pressure, and high cholesterol, among other challenges, can be at least partially improved with a better lifestyle, including regular exercise and a healthier diet.

The answer seems too simple, doesn't it? Diet and exercise: we often hear these two words together. Could the solution be more obvious?

It is so easy to fall for a quick fix, short-term, or temporary solution to our problem. The liquid diet, get in shape with ten minutes of working out a week, take this pill to have total control over the food—the list can go on! In the end, it all comes back to—you guessed it—proper diet and moderate exercise!

Attack your bad eating behavior with both the spiritual and the physical sides. In doing so, you will pull the deeper problems up by the root and address them directly. You will also create a healthy eating structure for yourselves at the same time. The fruits of your labor will be weight loss and long-term weight maintenance as a result of your work on the deeper problems.

QUESTIONS

- What does your "bed" look like for you at this moment?

- List one change you would like to see in your life. How can you go about changing this? What will you do to see this change happen? Be sure to give yourself credit for what you do or what you have that is good and worthy of maintaining.

For example, if you want more confidence, you can hire a professional wardrobe consultant to help you choose styles that are right for your body. If you want to get out of isolated eating habits, you can plan your evenings in advance and look forward to activities that will get you out of the house.

To summarize, poor eating habits are often a result of three things:

- Unresolved problems you have not dealt with, which indirectly manifest themselves in bad eating behavior
- A lack of understanding about nutrition
- A lack of an effective eating structure

VALUES *VS.* IDEALS

A **value** is a benefit we recognize as good and worthwhile, and we choose to possess it now by sacrificing other things. In contrast, an **ideal** is something we regard as beneficial and rewarding, and we want to have it in our life sometime in the future, but we are unwilling to relinquish for it at this time.

HOMEWORK

On the following Values vs. Ideals Chart, Column #1 is a list of things you could value. If this is a value of yours, check it in Column #2. In Column #3, look at the activities or habits you checked as values. Indicate how much time you have spent in the last month pursuing this value with A (a lot of time), B (a little time) or C (no time at all).

COLUMN #1	COLUMN #2	COLUMN #3
Activity or Habit	**Is this a value of yours?**	**A = Most days** **B = Sometimes** **C = Not much**
Regular exercise		
Worthwhile reading		
Mindless activities (surfing the net, computer games)		
Planning a healthy diet		
Smoking or drinking		
Staying within your budget		
Devotional or quiet time		
Time with friends or family		

Did you check *planning healthy diet* and *regular exercise* as values, yet your answer in Column #3 was C? If so, these are ideals for you and not values. Go through the chart and be realistic. Have you gotten values confused with ideals?

Some people say that eating healthfully is a value, yet they regularly make poor choices in restaurants and in the grocery store. They often eat junk food late at night and frequently skip meals. For them, eating better is an ideal, but they are not spending time creating a healthy diet in their lives. If they actually spent time working toward this goal, it would become a reality.

Strong values are defended intensely, whereas weaker values are more easily compromised. However, you can always choose to change your behavior.

QUESTIONS

- Have you denied yourself a lifestyle of healthy diet and regular exercise?

- Have you replaced it with a trendy "Lose Weight Fast!" solution that is here today and gone tomorrow?

- In your journal, write about an example of how you have avoided the truth. Some ways we do this are with rationalization, excuses, or an unwillingness to do what we know we need to do.

HOMEWORK

Are you ready to accept the simple solution of a healthy diet and regular exercise? Can you begin to apply it and work it into your lifestyle? In your journal, list one thing you can begin to do today—something to improve your lifestyle regarding food and physical activity. Date your entry, mark it on your calendar, and check it off each day. Continue to do this one thing for the next twenty-one days to make this a habit. Your choice could be something as simple as walking twenty minutes a day, drinking a glass of water with meals, or meditating ten minutes each morning.

After the three weeks are over, assess where you are with your efforts to change this one habit. How consistent were you? Do you feel better about yourself? Has your motivation increased? Have you done well? If so, add one more change in addition to maintaining the first. Do this for twenty-one more days. Continue with this pattern. Before you know it, self-improvement will be a habit. You will be living differently.

MORE QUESTIONS

Do you want to depend on the medical system for your health? Do you want to tote a bag of pills with you each day for your physical "imbalances?"

Or, do you want to take more control of your situation by doing the things you know would be healthy for you? What medical conditions do you have right now? Do you have some issues that may be reversible through lifestyle adjustments? Can you alter your behavior to make these changes? If so, what are you waiting for? What is holding you back?

Many reading this might be unwilling to make lifestyle changes. They may assume the pills will do all the work. Some take cholesterol-lowering drugs to substitute for eating junky food and being a couch potato, or inject themselves with insulin so they can eat huge desserts. The truth is the medicine is supposed to work in *conjunction* with the patient's behavioral changes, not compensate for them.

Some people still will not change their behavior even after they face a serious problem. They may be diagnosed with any number of overweight/inactivity-related diseases, such as diabetes, heart disease, gout, edema, or high blood pressure. These issues are not always connected to poor lifestyle, but in many cases, they are.

JUDY'S STORY

Judy was a loyal, long-term client of mine. She knew most of the results she sought would be up to her. She was determined to have consistent attendance, eat a light meal before her sessions, and get plenty of sleep the night before our appointments.

Like many clients seeking better health, Judy had high cholesterol and took prescription drugs to lower it. She believed her excess weight was partly to blame for her health issue, and losing this weight was one of her goals. Another goal was to be pill-free. Now, this is a loftier goal than simply losing weight. Her ambitions would require approval from her doctor. Judy had an idea.

She had an appointment with her physician to measure her numbers, and she asked him to lower her meds. She was surprised at the resistance she received from him. In fact, if she hadn't pushed to decrease the medicine, her doctor never would have adjusted it. However, she made a deal. She asked to have the medication lowered at that time. At their next appointment, if the numbers weren't better, the original dose would once again be prescribed. The doctor agreed.

This put Judy on the spot. She had something specific to work toward and a timeline—*both are important things one must have to set and successfully reach a goal.*

Judy did it. She lost the weight, and in doing so, her cholesterol dropped to a healthy level. The numbers convinced her doctor to lower the medicine. This process went on for some time. Eventually, she was no longer taking any drugs for cholesterol.

FINAL THOUGHTS

I'm so glad you don't have to be counted among those who depend entirely on medicine to keep you healthy. Rather, you are seeking positive solutions. You are not relying on a doctor to prescribe a solution for you. You are changing your choices and taking control of your life.

And this is empowering.

You now have the ability to arm yourself with the truth. This is the first step in moving forward with your life and seeing permanent change occur with your eating behavior.

There is no easy way around the truth. No pill will fix the problem, no weight loss diet with special food, and no passive exercise will achieve firm abs.

Let's quit looking elsewhere for the answer. It has already arrived. And we have found it.

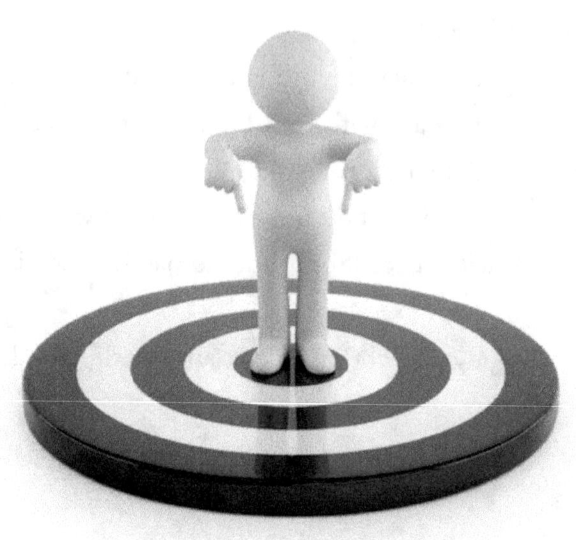

7. SETTING GOALS

"All improvement is dependent upon you seeing yourself as being greater than you are. Then your potentials stir within you and your creative capacities unfold. By your own inner self, you are led aright, and you glimpse the you that you are going to be." —Raymond Charles Barker

You will achieve when you set goals. You'll get nowhere if you don't. Do you know specifically what you want? Do you want to run a marathon, go on an African safari, lose ten pounds, climb Mount Everest, or get your degree? Have you made a plan toward this? Are you working each day to attain it? If you aren't specific about your target, it will be impossible to achieve it. This section will show you how to set good, realistic goals and create direction for your life.

Setting goals is as easy as 1-2-3. The first requirement is to be as specific as possible about what you want. Do you have a certain amount you want to weigh? How about a particular dress size you want to be? Or maybe you want to fit into some jeans you haven't worn in a long time? You need to be realistic with this goal, so don't set yourself up for failure. Make sure it is attainable.

This is the first thing you'll do. In your journal, set aside a separate section for goals. You will often refer to these pages and modify them as you go along. Goal-setting will become a part of your life, focused on where you want to go.

In your journal, set aside a separate section for goals.

The second item is to set a timeline. When do you want your goal attained? You need this deadline to motivate you. Be pragmatic in your expectations. If it's too soon, you might get discouraged and quit. Too distant will demotivate you. If you are unsure about what is reasonable, ask someone or research the topic.

Third, make a practical plan for attaining your goal. Set daily, weekly, and monthly plans. Break down the big achievements into smaller, easier goals. Be certain to do at least one thing every day.

It's important to write your ideas down so they will be embedded in your subconscious. Record your goals, and recall them daily. This will have a profound, motivating force in your life. If you don't believe me, do it anyway. You'll see that it works. So take some time now with your journal, and write out the three steps above to attain your goals. Look at them daily to measure your progress.

Reaching a goal can be tricky business. Unexpected things get in the way, and you'll need to make adjustments. Stay on track anyway!

Often, past experiences keep you in unhealthy patterns of behavior. It may take some soul searching to discover the roots of these roadblocks. Only then will you be able to become the person you want to be—emotionally and physically.

Are you excited about reaching your goals? I am excited for you! So how will you start? **Make that list now!**

CLARA'S STORY

Most of her life, Clara felt insecure and had no confidence. Her family moved frequently, and she didn't have close friends. She also had many siblings, so she didn't get attention from her parents. What she did receive was negative.

From her mother, Clara learned that men were interested in sex and nothing else. She also learned to loathe her own sexuality and dislike her body and its uniqueness. From her father, Clara learned that women are for men to look at and appreciate, but they must never get angry or speak their minds.

Furthermore, she learned from her father that women are inferior, and never smarter than men. All of these messages played a part in destroying Clara's self-confidence. They also affected Clara's outlook on life and her behavior with food. She overate as a reaction to these unhealthy ideas.

When Clara was a teenager, she started to gain weight. Then she became so concerned with being the perfect size, she went on regular crash diets. If she were skinny, she thought, she wouldn't have any problems. She felt empty and directionless, living for years by the false messages of her parents. She attempted to stuff down her emptiness and uncomfortable emotions with food. People, places, and things made her scared or fearful, so she avoided new experiences.

Clara used the food in place of a more abundant life. She avoided taking risks. When she eventually lost complete control over her food, her weight climbed. Desperate, she didn't realize her unpleasant childhood still impacted her.

Once she realized she was in a bad place, she became teachable and open-minded. Surfing the internet one day, she found how some people had successfully lost weight through self-awareness. She embarked on her own path of self-examination and found her problem. Her issues weren't about food: Clara simply didn't like Clara. She didn't have a food problem; she had a *living* problem.

Becoming aware of these messages was the first step toward her permanent weight loss. She went through the uncomfortable process of journaling into her past and becoming aware of her dysfunctional childhood. She eventually understood the reasons for her poor choices. The revelation changed her life.

Once she knew where her behavior originated, she had a choice. She could continue to act in the old ways, or she could take charge of her life. Determined to exert her power of control over her own life, she began to react differently to life's situations.

As a result of her introspective work, Clara lost weight and has kept it off permanently.

QUESTIONS

Did you receive unhealthy messages from your parents when you were a child? Have these affected you negatively? Write the name of each parent or guardian on a separate sheet of paper. Consider how their behavior toward you has impacted you. Freely journal about your feelings, and be open to discovering new insights. These nuggets of truth can give you both direction and the freedom to make different choices in the future.

Do you owe any of your parents an apology? Do you need to communicate to them? Has there been a long silence between you? If you realize you should initiate reconciliation and you take the steps to do so, you will grow in maturity. Don't let pride keep you from becoming a better person. Holding on to past grievances can only hurt you.

Reflecting on Clara's story, are there any messages you learned early in life that you continue to respond to by overeating?

MORE QUESTIONS

How do you react to unpleasant circumstances in life? Reflect on the past week, and record a time you felt especially agitated. Record what the event was. Then, record what effect the event had on you emotionally. In other words, how you internally processed the event—if you snapped at someone or if you overate as a result. Finally, record how significant the event actually was, or if it was only a minor irritation.

Answering these questions will identify the difference between your reaction to an event and its significance. Is your response appropriate? This self-examination will help you alter the way you process events that cause inner tension.

Do the short-lived problems cause as much stress in the moment as the longer-term problems? Are there any differences in your reactions? Become aware of how your body and stress level respond to different types of stress, and pay attention to how you may react. You can even start a log of each event to record your progress.

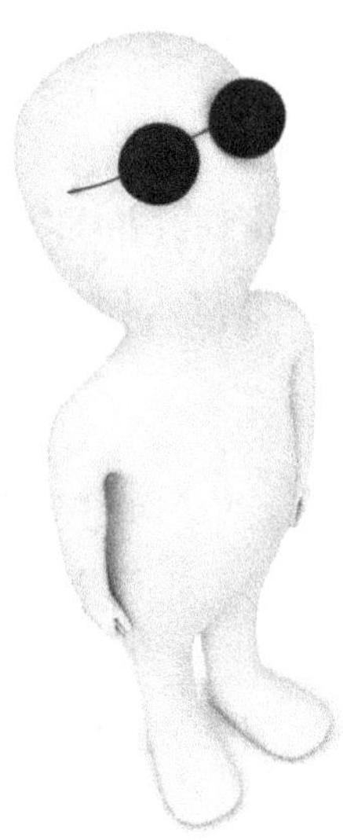

8. CHANGE YOUR FOCUS!

"The secret of change is to focus all of your energy, not on fighting the old, but on building the new." —Socrates

Most overweight people focus on their excess pounds as the cause of their problems, when other things might be responsible for their unhappiness.

I recommend a different approach: start to change yourself by focusing on undesirable areas of your character. This will focus your energy from food toward attaining a better "you," and will shift your attention off the food and onto your personality. In doing so, you will discover your weight-loss formula.

When you begin to move toward self-improvement, you will change your overall lifestyle for the better. **You** are the one who discovers what needs to be changed. **You** are the one who decides how to go about making these changes. **You** maintain total control over the process. No one is telling you what you should do—you are using your intuition to find the answers you seek!

You are using your intuition to find the answers you seek.

Weight loss can certainly be a by-product of your efforts toward self-improvement. In most cases, it happens naturally. This may seem counter-intuitive at first, but if you try it for a few weeks, you'll see a profound difference in your mental attitude and your eating habits.

Let's change our focus and start working on the seemingly unimportant and/or minor things—those easy to brush off and ignore. Don't try to get your eating right before you address your bad habits. Correcting your food may be a matter of resolving these issues first. In fact, losing weight may be contingent upon this. In any case, you can't go wrong by digging a bit and gaining some self-understanding.

Consider how a prism works. The prism refracts the light, dividing it into the colors of the visible spectrum. Red, orange, yellow, green, blue, indigo, and violet: all are seen. And with a single prism, you get all these. There is no picking and choosing which colors come through.

You are a complete person, interconnected in every way possible. Nothing you do, say, or feel is compartmentalized. Everything affects your mind and body in ways you may not know. Start today by looking at yourself like you would a prism. Visualize all your actions and feelings (individual colors) and their impact on your life (the complete rainbow).

However, I am not saying to continue eating junk food or bingeing while you work on these other aspects of your life. Such behavior would be futile. Suppose you were to continue your bad food habits while trying to improve other areas of your life. Your efforts to improve one area and not the other would create two competing and opposite forces inside you, one positive and the other negative. Unfortunately, the negative side is bound to gain more strength, and you will be back where you started from, if not worse.

Recall this part of Abraham Lincoln's speech on June 16, 1858, "A house divided against itself cannot stand. I believe this government cannot endure, permanently, half slave and half free." Going further back in history, in Matthew 12:25, Jesus says, "…*Every kingdom divided against itself will be ruined, and every city or household divided against itself will not stand.*"

If you tackle some issues you see need improvement, yet leave others untouched, you are bound to fail. The negativity you've fallen into has too much momentum, is too strong, and is too deeply entrenched. What I am really talking about is an attitude adjustment.

Let's look at this a different way. Imagine your whole being looks like an onion—that's right: an onion. When you buy one from the store, it has a thick, hardened, or crusty exterior. We don't like to eat that part, because the good part is the tender meat on the inside. How many layers of the onion do you need to discard before reaching the edible portion?

If you are this onion, then how many layers do you need to remove to find the real "you?" Do you have to cry some tears to get closer to the inside? How does removing one layer of "skin" impact other areas of your life?

If you remove a single piece of skin, the whole onion is bared a little bit. As more layers are removed, the tender and desirable part is more exposed. Likewise, as you grow mature, others will perceive you as approachable and authentic. You will feel a greater connection to humanity, and fear of people will leave you.

Develop a mindset to work *both* the food and the character improvement at the same time, but spend most of your energy on internal development. Don't get too dismayed when you fail with your food one day. Pick yourself back up, continue on, and focus on some positive action you can take unrelated to diet. A positive mindset is required for worthy and lasting change.

A positive mindset is required
for worthy and lasting change.

HOMEWORK

Make a list of several daily things you would like to improve. These might include items for you to do in order to create a fresh viewpoint. Something simple could include an action, such as cleaning the hairbrush after you use it, cleaning the drain after you finish showering, changing the toilet paper rolls when they are empty, making your bed as soon as you get up in the morning, or putting your dishes in the dishwasher instead of leaving them in the sink.

Some other things could be spending ten minutes in meditation a day, always unloading the dishwasher or dryer (instead of waiting for someone else to do it), allowing the other driver to enter in front of you, or leaving five minutes earlier for appointments to guarantee punctuality. If you are a tactile person, keep your hands busy with productive and/or creative activities.

What action could you take to improve your relationship with someone you love? Can you think of something you could change that matters to that person, and would make them feel loved?

If you wake up one day in a negative state of mind, force yourself to focus on things you enjoy. Take your list of goals, and start doing something toward each one of them. Don't stop until you have attained a happier outlook. You will see definite, ongoing improvement in your life through your positive actions. Also, you will be more likely to stick with your food plan if your mind and emotions are in the right place.

DAVID'S STORY

David thought that if he only knew why he ate so much, he would have the power to stop overeating. He believed this awareness was the answer to his food problem. He stayed stuck in this mindset for years. He continued to eat, remained overweight, and believed the lie that all he needed to know was the reason why he ate.

David put the cart before the horse. Conquering food addiction works the other way around. He had to first quit abusing the food, and *then* he could see why he had been overeating. The only way he could lose weight and keep it off would be for him to let go of the excessive food—for an extended period—and substitute better actions.

His full-time work preoccupied his mind, and food did not pose a problem. The free and unstructured time proved his challenge. As a single man living alone, isolation became a natural by-product of his lifestyle, and indulging in excess food followed.

To succeed in losing weight, he had to stay out of the kitchen between meals. When he did this, suddenly he had a lot more time. This was a revelation to him—the amount of time he wasted eating unneeded food.

He began to substitute his bad habit with a more healthy and rewarding one—talking on the phone. He made a quick list of a dozen names of friends and family he could call, just to chat. He called his buddies from college and his two brothers, his parents, his cousin, and a group of friends from church. Usually, he could find someone to talk with.

Those few moments were all it took to make the cravings go away!

Obviously, he found a solution to his problem. Deepening his close relationships satisfied an unrecognized need for friendships and dissolved his cravings to overeat.

So how can *you* put the food down? How can you stop overeating and start doing something different? What are you supposed to do as a substitute? Even then, will it be sufficient so the desire for excess food dwindles away?

You can't succeed in any endeavor inside a vacuum. You can't eliminate a bad habit outright, and expect it to stay away. If you want lasting change, you must find an adequate form of compensation for what you need to give up. This is the only logical way toward sustainability.

> **If you want lasting change, you must find an adequate form of compensation for what you need to give up.**

And this is exactly what I want you to find—a substitute for the food that will more than compensate you for what you initially got from all that excess eating. So continue to read and discover your process to develop your individual formula for success.

I want to mention two things here. First, substitutes for bad habits require a certain period of readjustment. Don't expect your food cravings or compulsions to overeat to leave immediately. In fact, expect them to resist your efforts to change. Make plans to respond aggressively with constructive action. This will directly combat those negative drives in you and will help you overcome them sooner. Tools for healthy living are found in the last section of the book. Here, you will be given helpful suggestions to assist your transition to a healthier lifestyle.

Second, any kind of change you initiate will involve some degree of faith. You might know what you want to do, and are willing to make it a goal. You probably won't know what your lifestyle will look like once you get there. However, all change is uncomfortable—you can count on that. And looking forward, how can you be sure you will like the change?

Something surprised me once I embarked on this new lifestyle of self-examination. For the first month or two, I actually *grieved* the loss of my bad eating habits. It was true sadness, as if a companion had died—and it had, although this wasn't a true friend. I had no idea I would face this flood of negative emotions, but since I had made my decision to live differently, I accepted the grief as part of the process. Eventually, it left me, and I realized I'd lost an enemy, rather than a friend.

The best advice I can give here is don't project into the future and create a mindset of fear. If you do, you might convince yourself it's not even worth attempting. Keep your focus steady and move forward with what you know you want—a healthier, leaner body, and better eating habits.

To summarize, a change you invoke in your own life will involve some unknown factors. You will need to cultivate a feeling of "comfortable-ness" with these unknowns and get used to not knowing everything about the future. You know you don't want to continue on your present road, and you are ready to get off. As you work the written drills, journal, and begin to know yourself better, you will have a clearer picture of where your path will lead you.

LOTTIE'S STORY

When Lottie was in junior high school, she had control over her eating. She could gradually cut back her food to lose a little weight without becoming obsessed with the whole diet/weight loss thing, but the fact she had to cut back to lose weight was an indication she already had a problem manifesting.

When she was in her freshman year of high school, she began fasting for several days to lose weight quickly. She broke those fasts by eating sacks of candy.

Somewhere during her teenage years, she transitioned from casual, unconscious eating to bingeing. She became obsessed with her weight. Her food and appearance became her primary focus, controlling every part of her life to the point of obsession. "If only I could fix my food, then I would be happy," was her mantra.

During this season of her life, she ate things that didn't even taste good to her, and ate more than she really wanted. Her body cried, "Stop, please stop!" Yet she kept on eating and lost all boundaries with food. "Anything goes, and nothing works." She had no discipline, no absolutes, and no fixed eating schedule. With such a lack of structure, it was impossible for her to get on track. She became a yo-yo dieter.

For Lottie, her solution involved achieving some self-discipline. She also needed a sound nutritional diet to give her body what it needed, regularly.

For self-discipline, the fasting had to stop, and the candy binges had to stop. This cycle almost drove her crazy and made her more obsessed. Also, for her to find a sound diet schedule, she needed a little assistance from a qualified nutrition professional.

Her advisor had a powerful impact on her. She gave Lottie the appropriate information to help make the best nutritional choices for her body. An added benefit was accountability. She had to schedule regular appointments, record her food in a journal, and follow up. All these actions took several months and helped her to develop positive habits for lasting change.

QUESTIONS

1. Do you remember a time when you had control over your food choices, but no longer have it? When did this happen? If not, do you feel threatened you may lose control?
2. Do you sometimes binge, then return to normal eating?

3. What do you do when unwanted and tempting food comes into your home?
4. Where is your downfall, your weak spot?
5. Can you list some alternatives to or substitutes for unhealthy eating?
6. Are you ready to begin?

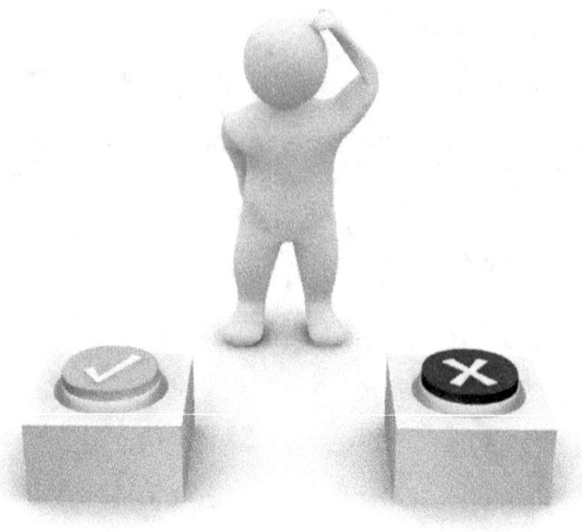

9. THREE CONTINUUMS

"Admit that your own private Mount Everest exists. That is half the battle." —Hugh Macleod

A continuum is a two-dimensional graph with opposites on either end. In this section, I use them to help you get an idea of where you are.

When you began reading this book, you most likely had a goal to lose weight. Since then, you have come to realize there is more to the excess weight than a few pounds. You learned there is internal work to accomplish. Now, the next step is to decide where you stand on certain issues. Doing so will help you determine the work you need to do to insure permanent weight loss.

If you have tried really hard to lose weight, yet you are still overweight and stuck on old behaviors, consider this: gain insight through introspection. Self-honesty and journaling about anything that bothers you could work wonders for you.

FROM STRESS TO PEACE

Eating as a result of stress in our lives is a huge cause of our excess weight. Anxiety can be internal or external. It can be self-inflicted, imaginary, intentionally brought upon us by others, or haphazardly wreaked on us (think traffic jam).

Sometimes unresolved issues from our past, either recent or long ago, hover over us constantly and prevent us from becoming the whole, healthy person we were created to be. We may become accustomed to this dark cloud of trepidation until we can imagine nothing else. Unable to relax and find peace in our lives, we develop a victim mindset and believe constant tension is normal.

What is the solution? Your habitual reaction—unhealthy eating—doesn't help! A better answer is to uncover the origin of your pressure and decide how to respond to it in a healthier way. Train yourself to live differently, become open minded to self-examination. Become tuned-in with your emotions, and learn to respond in ways that honor yourself. This can take a lifetime and still not be perfected, but it is the most effective approach for us problem-eaters.

A few bites of food may give you a moment's relief from your difficulty, and you may believe you are still in control. However, until you uncover the source and deal with the cause of your overeating, you will likely fall back into your old patterns of food abuse. You may become totally discouraged and feel you will never find permanent results.

Become open-minded to self-examination.

Find your formula by exploring all possibilities that may seem unimportant or even unrelated to the food. You may be surprised at what you uncover during this "fact finding mission," but if you make a start and see the results of your efforts, I am certain you will be sold on this way of life.

Since there are different types of aggravations, and since each one of us responds differently, each has to be dealt with and tailored to you as an individual. Here again, I want to emphasize the reason why most diet plans don't work. *They don't get to the roots of problems.* Rather, they only stay on the surface and focus on the types of food and quantities to eat.

Uncovering your burdens is not as hard as it sounds. One of the things you can begin to do is to reach out to trusted friends or professionals for information on how to deal with specific situations. Explore your questions with individuals you trust. Go with your instinct, and let it lead you to the counsel you need.

For example, if you feel totally lost about your life's direction, you may want to consult a therapist or life coach. If you are confused about all the conflicting information surrounding fat, sugar, and nutrition in general, you may consider talking with a nutritionist. Finally, if you just need to bounce things off someone, why don't you schedule a regular coffee or walk with a friend?

CARRIE'S STORY

Carrie grew up thinking that her parents and siblings were A-1, tops, "best friends," always to be trusted. When her life began to change and she started implementing the ideas in this book, she quickly realized her family members were not the best confidants. When she shared with one of her sisters, her secrets were repeated to another sister, breaking her confidence.

Through this experience, Carrie became wiser. The hurt feelings she experienced motivated her to trust her feelings, relying only on those who truly support her. Once she came to this realization and accepted it, she was able to move on. She no longer wasted her time trying to make someone something they weren't, even a family member.

QUESTIONS

- Where would you place yourself on the Stress-Peace Continuum?
- What can you do today to move yourself closer to inner peace?

If something causes stress, try to deal with it effectively. If nothing can be done about it, leave it alone and accept it the way it is. You might get temporary "comfort" from eating a sleeve of crackers with block of cheese (or whatever snack food you choose), but the next day you probably wouldn't feel too good about yourself, so this would—in actuality—result in more stress. Find and follow things that create peace within you.

Before you take that first bite, check your emotional state. Are you feeling frustrated, angry, depressed, or any combination of negative emotions? These feelings may be precursors to unhealthy eating habits.

Try to practice detaching your emotions from your eating. Instead, shift your focus from immediate gratification to delayed gratification and long-term peace. Instead of looking at the initial satisfaction from eating something (and the stress-relief it seems to provide), look at everything you'll get from eating that food. It may not seem so attractive after all.

FROM ABUSE TO NURTURE

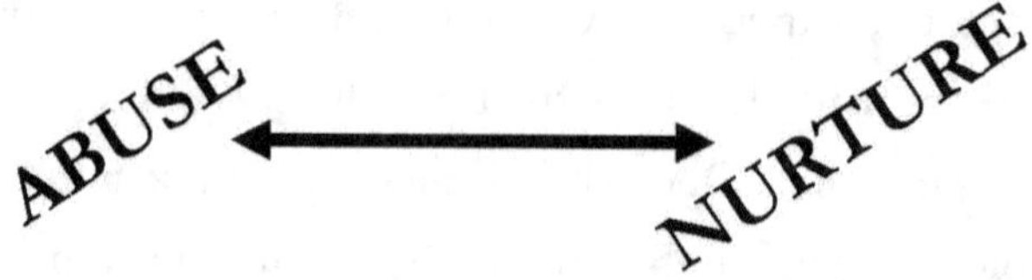

Webster defines abuse as, to "use improperly or injuriously; misuse." That definition is pretty broad, but it leads me to the question, "what does abusing *food* mean?"

We can all agree that the purpose of food is to nurture our physical health. However, if we examine our eating habits, we find a great deal of our behavior is unhealthy and will actually harm our bodies. We can admit we use food for reasons other than to sustain life. Again, this is very basic, but I am trying to make a comparison between the purpose of food and our varied uses (and abuses) of it.

I think we can all say that at some point we have abused food to some degree. What about Thanksgiving dinner or the holidays? This is almost a universal excuse for overeating and abusing food. Everybody is doing it, so it's okay, right? Or what about eating at a restaurant? You're full, yet you continue to eat because you enjoy it so much. And for those who've been on a cruise, have you noticed how you indulge?

It's easy to rationalize overdoing something so prevalent, especially when we see others doing the same thing. It makes us feel more comfortable. We even see chubby movie stars and other role models, and it seems like the new "normal." It is definitely more socially acceptable these days. This is a good thing, because everybody needs acceptance, whether fat or not. But is the behavior and the excess weight right for *you*?

Some plump individuals seem to be happy, unconcerned about their weight. Some heavy individuals may even proclaim their super-sized physique makes them happy. Furthermore, people have made successful careers based on their obesity. Is it any of our business? And does their claim to be a happy fat person make us feel happier about our excess weight?

If you have a tendency to rationalize your actions based upon what someone else's life looks like, you must stop that behavior right now! We need to get our feelings of self-confidence from inside us, rather than judging ourselves by what others are saying or doing.

HOMEWORK

Visualize the person you want to be. Is that person thin? Does that person smile and laugh often? Does that person think often of others? Try to get a clear mental picture of this person and recall this vision as often as possible.

NICK'S STORY

Using food for comfort, Nick isolated himself at home. Food was a convenient activity when he was frustrated or stressed. It took on an identity in itself, and began to dominate him. Not even realizing the impact his behavior had, a clandestine affair with excess food resulted. Shame ensued. And for years, this relationship was the substitute for human friendships.

His relationships with others were superficial or work-related. Food was more of a priority for him. He ate when he needed to and even when he didn't, simply because of habit. Whenever he felt emotional tension, eating was the panacea.

He developed a habit of constant hand-to-mouth eating that seemed to comfort his emotional hunger for human friendships. Shy and fearful of approaching others, he did not know how to initiate a conversation, so he kept on eating to avoid relationships.

The food's true purpose became distorted in his mind and in his emotions. Through counseling, journaling, and self-examination, Nick recognized his abusive behavior and gained insight into his deep-rooted fear of socializing.

He'd always loved cycling, so he connected with a local bicycle club. This indirect way to associate with others didn't require anything other than his attendance. This helped him shift from food abuse to a more nurturing lifestyle. He faced his fear, and forced himself to talk to people he met on bike rides. These friendships blossomed into other social activities. Eventually, he left his bad eating habits behind him, and began to nurture himself by eating properly and moderately. At the same time, he increased participation in his cycling club, and the exercise helped him to drop more pounds.

When he got connected with others, the hunger he originally tried to fill with food was satisfied with human relationships. He didn't need excess food anymore.

QUESTIONS

- Where would you place yourself on the Abuse-Nurture Continuum?
- How can you shift your eating habits to be more nurturing and less abusing?
- How much of your eating results from an abusive place versus a nurturing place?
- Considering Nick's story, do you have any unrecognized fears?

No food tastes as good as healthy living feels!

We can always find room for improvement. Maybe it's losing that last five pounds, eating more vegetables, getting off sugar, or exercising more. So remember: no food tastes as good as healthy living feels.

Again, the proper purpose for food is primarily to sustain life, and then for enjoyment. However, if our health is at risk, we may not be able to afford the luxury of eating for enjoyment anymore—at least not at every meal.

Make the decision to begin taking better care of your body and your mind by exploring your real hungers and treating yourself as well as possible.

FROM ENTITLEMENT TO SELF-HONESTY

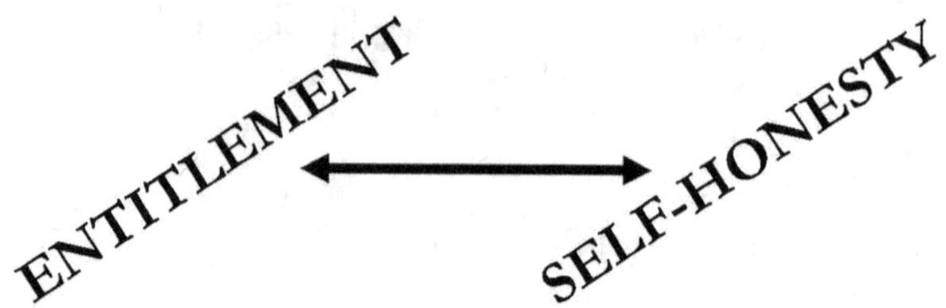

"*I deserve to reward myself because I've had such a bad day.*" Have you had similar thoughts, and proceeded to comfort yourself with food? How did you feel afterwards? How about the next day? Did you try not to think about it, yet still had a nagging feeling about having failed at your diet one more day? If your self-honesty got you this far, did you convince yourself you were hopeless and would never succeed so why try anyway? Might as well eat what I want today also. I'm already fat, so a little more eating won't be noticeable on my body. What's the use?

In the paragraph above, suppose this person is you. Your weight and eating habits are a problem, and you indulged as a result of an event or string of occurrences. Tell me where the problem originated. Did it start when the thing that caused your bad day occurred? Did it evolve from your rationalization you deserve to reward yourself? Did it begin when you took the first bite? Or did it have anything to do with a hangover of negative thoughts from the previous day?

Let's look at each one of the above questions and gain insight.

Question 1: Did it start when the thing that caused your bad day occurred? Bad event(s) in anyone's life are never an excuse to eat. Life is all about facing challenging situations. How you decide to respond to these is your challenge. You can go through life and react by abusing food, or you can decide to make different choices.

Question 2: Did it evolve from the rationalization you deserve to reward yourself? At this point, we process a circumstance and choose to internalize it or not. Our problem starts in our mind and how we choose to think. We can go one way or another. If we choose the unhealthy foods, we have made a bad choice. However, since we can change our choices, we can change our responses. The place to make the change is inside our heads, as we process a problem.

Question 3: Did it begin when you took the first bite? This action is the result of the problem, and not the core issue itself. It is the result of improper thinking, poor choices, and possibly a negative mindset. The thoughts are the roots and must be removed from the soil of your mind. Get your hand around the noxious bulb buried in your thoughts, and yank it out.

Question 4: Did it have anything to do with a hangover of negative thoughts from the previous day? Your thinking plays the most powerful part in your success with any endeavor. If you begin a day with a negative mindset, you are more likely to fail than to succeed with any goal. Begin each day with conscious intention to maintain a positive outlook. Discipline your mind to see beauty. Carry a notebook with you, notice little things you are grateful for, and record these observations. The more you focus on these things, the bigger they get, and the negativity (and bad eating habits) will become a thing of the past.

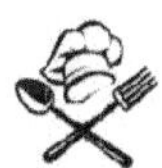

HOMEWORK

Focus on a recent time when you ate too much. Were you using the food to provide you with something food is not capable of satisfying, such as comfort, relaxation, or relationship?

Did you have expectations the food would solve the emotional issue you faced? If so, you might be subconsciously demanding overeating provide something it was never meant to provide. You might feel "entitled" to receive or get something that was never meant to be yours in the first place (at least not through these means). When you didn't properly address your challenge, you decided to overeat instead, to compensate for it.

Or maybe the entitlement was simply focused on taking more than you needed. Let's look at some possibilities with an open mind, and see if we might gain self-honesty.

> You might be subconsciously demanding overeating provide something it was never meant to provide.

LIZ'S STORY

Liz had a problem of trying to force her "square peg" self in to a "round hole" place, thinking if she only pushed hard enough, she could make herself fit.

She had a high-pressure job and wanted to excel in her profession, but for the wrong reasons. She wanted others to recognize her and pat her on the back so she would feel good about herself, but she could never get enough positive reinforcement from others.

She really didn't like her job at all or even the people from whom she sought approval. In forcing herself to stay, she refused to be honest with herself and constantly tried to make herself be someone else. She refused to accept her need for a different environment. She was simply not acknowledging herself for who she was.

Liz had been trying to live someone else's life. She thought conforming to her company's culture and schmoozing was going to make her successful. She believed she might gain the affirmation of others if she was successful.

In Liz's attempts to find this recognition, she was not being honest with herself. Her overeating became a habit to compensate for this self-dishonesty, and she consequently developed her problem with food.

An expected promotion was given to someone else, and her own angry reaction woke her up. She admitted she didn't like her job or the people in the company she worked for. She realized she sought approval from others when she should seek it from herself. She went on a job search, secured one in another industry she really loved, and left her company. Even though she took a pay cut, she was happy about her decision. She started to accept herself for who she was, and she lost her excess weight.

KEN'S STORY

Ken had been overweight most of his life. Food, eating, and yo-yo dieting were all longstanding habits with him. He was a master at denial and hated confrontation with anyone on any level. He finally reached a crisis in his life he couldn't avoid. This got his attention and forced him to seek counsel.

Excited to learn the unhealthy ways he dealt with life, Ken delved in to the dark crevices of his mind to enter a process of self-discovery, and he also obtained a food plan from a nutritionist that could fit into his lifestyle.

When he tackled both of these areas simultaneously, he realized why he ate so much and why he had abused food for so many years. He ate when things bothered him, rather than dealing immediately and directly with the irritations or the people who disturbed him.

Through the counseling process, Ken learned new ways to approach challenging circumstances. He began to identify specific feelings that preceded a binge, and to process those emotions as they arose. He no longer avoided them or stuffed them down with food. This time, the weight loss became permanent.

Here's the pattern of his overeating. (1) Any circumstance that created a (2) strong emotion—good, bad, exciting, sad, or frustrating—automatically caused a (3) physical craving for food. Once the desire to eat was there, in his mind the (4) rationalization entered and entitled him to (5) act accordingly.

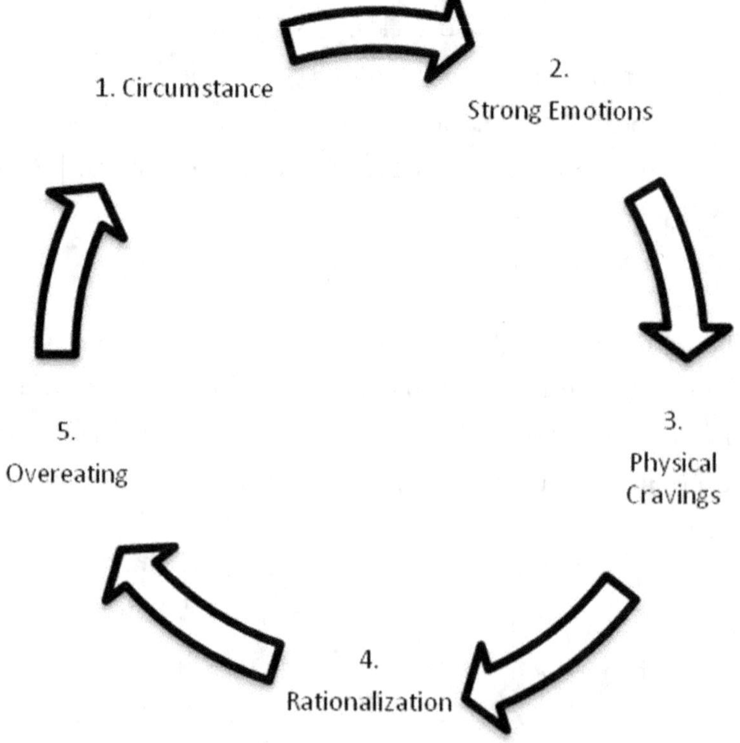

This cycle was how he dealt with everything in life. The more he lived this way, the stronger the cycle became. In fact, it got so strong the weight became his primary circumstance (back to (1) again). He became more focused on the weight than on other problems. The cycle didn't end with (5), but recycled back to (1) with greater vengeance than before.

This point is where many lose perspective on what key issues are challenges in their lives. They shift focus from a situation they could tackle constructively, and they wind up creating a problem on top of the other one. This makes it harder to unravel the issues to get to the core circumstances that caused our overeating in the first place.

Denial is a convenient way to evade problems, but it actually masks them and makes them harder to identify. Ken concentrated on the symptom, rather than the real issues.

> ## Denial is a convenient way to evade problems, but it actually masks them and makes them harder to identify.

Once he was deceived into believing all he needed to do was lose excess pounds, he was unable to do so because he lost his focus on the root of his weight gain. This created even more strong emotions, and he ate over his inability to control his eating. The cycle perpetuated itself.

Ken had to work his way backwards to the origin of his problem and find his warning signals of trouble. At first, he would realize when he was falling into a binge. Then, he became aware of his rationalization and worked at correcting his thinking. He knew he didn't want to eat. Nevertheless, this still did not give him immunity from overeating.

The next step was to harness his thoughts as they occurred and when external stimuli happened. He needed to become aware of subconscious reactions and eliminate them. He learned how to respond in healthy ways, rather than being driven by reflex.

The final step was to address his desire for food, connect that to the physical cravings, and see how a circumstance triggered the strong emotions and compulsion to eat. This took time and patience, but with perseverance, he finally succeeded.

Today, he has better control over his thoughts and catches them early in the cycle. This is a habit he acquired through counseling, and he continues to live this way today.

Can you imagine how happy he was to finally address the real problems? All that wasted time spent focusing on food, dieting, and losing weight, and the food really wasn't the problem: it was his internal responses.

HOMEWORK

Consider the cycle once again, as it applies to you. Recall a recent time when you were unhappy about your eating. Journal about the event, from start to finish. Draw the circle on a page in your journal. Determine where you entered each phase of the succession. What happened? What were you feeling? What was your self-talk? Was there a point of no return? Better yet, do you see a place where you could have stopped yourself in your self-destructiveness?

The cycle has five steps, from beginning to end. How long did it take for you to move through the process? Did one step take longer to go through than another? Examine all aspects of your event.

The more time you procrastinate from one phase of the cycle to another, the better your chances are of having a victory. Try to stretch out at least one stage the next time you catch yourself in this sequence. When you're stuck, make the distance longer and longer for each episode. If you can do this, your cravings are likely to leave you. You will be able to walk away from the food.

This activity is one that bears repeating multiple times before you succeed. Please persist, because even the smallest of victories can spawn hope and motivate you to try one more day.

I remember how ecstatic I was to have my first tiny victory. I wanted to shout out to the world! I had wrestled so long and was so tired, frustrated, and discouraged. The seemingly insignificant win didn't immediately drop eighty pounds of excess weight off my body, but I knew I was on my way. All I had to do was continue trying. I knew this was exactly what I needed for permanent weight loss in my future.

KRISTA'S STORY

Krista's boyfriend broke up with her for another woman. She felt rejected, angry, and depressed. Each day after work, she would go home, isolate herself for the rest of the evening, and binge on starchy, sugary foods. This went on for months, and the weight piled on. She wished she were motivated to eat right and work out, but felt overwhelmed at the thought.

Krista was a victim of *emotional constipation*. Her mental pipes were clogged with toxic, unaddressed emotions, and this polluted her life. She was unable to experience anything to its fullest. She was bogged down and mentally sluggish.

Determined to rid herself of these hindrances, she shared her feelings with a confidant. Her girlfriend asked if she had done any journaling about the break-up. She suggested Krista might be denying her anger toward her ex, burying her emotion with excess food. Could there be a few tears left to shed?

She admitted she hadn't done any self-examination. She did, however, acknowledge pain still remained, and took her pen to paper. Instead of her nightly binge routine, visits with her friend enabled her to process the break-up. The weight eventually came off.

SUMMARY

Is there something you need to write about, express on paper, and finally be done with? You can't process feelings by overeating—or any other unhealthy behavior. The only way to process something is to ask God for help, communicate your thoughts, and/or speak your mind. You can do this by meditating, journaling, or talking to a friend or therapist.

Do you think of your past actions as self-destructive? Yes, that's a strong idea. But do you at least admit your behavior has been essentially wrecking your life? Have you driven yourself to a point of no return? Slow or fast, have you decimated your chances for contentment with unaddressed buried emotions and inappropriate outward actions?

Do you think you have a choice in dealing with a problem or not? If you are a long-term sufferer of excess weight, you do not have this luxury. You must face issues, or you will self-destruct.

You must face issues, or you will self-destruct.

You thought we were finished with self-honesty? I'm here to tell you, it has only just begun. In fact, I will consider myself successful if you become more honest with food as well as other areas of your life.

Self-honesty is foundational. It shouldn't be confused with self-control, although they are related. Emotional restraint must come before self-discipline, although some of you reading this undoubtedly will have one but lack the other.

Some of you would probably like to stop overeating, but no matter what you do, the problem won't budge. For you, there may be a little more work involved to get to the bottom of why you can't control your eating at times.

Do you think you can handle this problem, but don't feel like addressing it right now? Don't fool yourself! The problem is destined to get worse with each passing day you avoid it. Success with your eating has to begin with self-honesty, regardless of whether or not you are an emotional eater or simply lack motivation.

Reluctance to sincerely look into yourself may perpetuate your bad situation and keep you from the triumph you truly wish for and deserve.

You need to honestly examine yourself, take ownership of how you feel and accept where you stand at this moment. Moving from that point, one step at a time, you will make suitable responses to your dilemmas. This will lead you toward peace and contentment.

Success with your eating has to begin with self-honesty, regardless of whether or not you are an emotional eater or simply lack motivation.

QUESTIONS

- Where are you in the 'Entitlement/Self-Honesty' Continuum?

- Is there something (or someone) in your life (or in your past) that you are trying to control?

- And what is your reaction to your not getting what you want: frustration, constant anger, depression, overeating, or something else?

HOMEWORK

Let's go through a little more self-diagnosis. Draw a horizontal line across a page in your journal. Place a 0 at the far left point and a 100 on the far right. Zero stands for absolutely no nutritional understanding, no motivation, and uncontrolled eating every day. One hundred stands for total nutritional mastery and awareness of where to obtain additional knowledge, total self-control, and good, consistent motivation— perfection.

0=No Nutritional Understanding or Motivation

100=Total Nutritional Mastery and Self-Control

Now, with regard to these things, where do you place yourself on this continuum? Obviously, no one will be zero or one hundred. Do you simply sometimes crave certain foods and succumb to the craving? Could you even go as far as to say you might be slightly or even very prone to unhealthy eating patterns? Or do you simply lack information, yet are motivated? By lacking information, I mean do you know exactly what to put in your mouth, how much, and when? Finally, do you have all the insight you need to get the results you want, yet are simply unmotivated?

ARE YOU READY TO CHANGE YOUR VIEW?

"When the student is ready, the teacher will appear." —Buddhist Proverb

I was raised to believe I could control my life, or at least believe I could fix anything that wasn't the way I wanted it to be.

When I was in Paris, I learned how wrong I was. When I realized my food and eating were out of control, that was the beginning of my being receptive to a different way of life and a new way of eating. But the bingeing went on for quite some time before I realized that my worldview had shattered. At this point, I became willing to listen to others' points of view. About that time, I found a weight-loss support group in the church.

If you know you are hooked into an unhealthy lifestyle and unable to pull yourself out of your rut, have you come to the realization that your attempts at control do not work anymore? Unless you've reached the limits of your own efforts, the principles in this book may not work as well for you.

Where will you be in five years from now if you continue as you are? What about ten years? What will your life look like then? How much might you weigh? How large will you be?

Perhaps you are young and don't have health complications as a result of your eating—yet. Maybe your energy is high and your joints are still strong enough to carry your body. You may think foot and knee problems are not yours, but they may loom in your near future. What about autoimmune diseases, heart disease, or diabetes?

Try to think of how your life could unravel, and decide now if your current lifestyle is the one you want in the years ahead. Are you ready to change?

I'm not trying to create a spirit of fear in you. Instead, I want you to predict where your bad habits will lead you. Be wise and take control now, while you can. Make bold decisions. Determine what you want your life to look like later on.

Predict where your bad habits will lead you.

You don't have to do this on your own. Many professionals can help you reach your goals. Some of you may need instruction, and others may need to seek more emotional support to stay focused.

If you need help selecting nutritional foods in the right combinations, hire a qualified nutritionist. If you eat as a result of stress, hire a life coach or counselor. If you need motivation to maintain your chosen level of fitness, hire a certified personal trainer.

I caution you to be proactive with these professionals. Don't plop down your money and expect them to "do it" for you! Unless you take possession of your goals, when the time for using these caregivers ends, you will be more vulnerable to reverting to your old ways.

You must take their information and integrate it into your own life. Ask questions, go to the gym on your own the days you don't see your trainer, and learn the equipment by yourself. Develop skills from counseling, and read food labels when you grocery shop. If you don't claim ownership of your life, who will?

A WORD ON MOTIVATION

Since you have stuck with me all this time, you must have at least a seed of motivation. Yes, this is the key! All you need is a little incentive. Nurture it, pay attention to it, and watch it grow. You are on your way. As you persevere, day by day and hour by hour, your motivation will grow. I'm proud of you for reading this far. By the way, we'll delve much deeper into motivation in a later section, so keep reading.

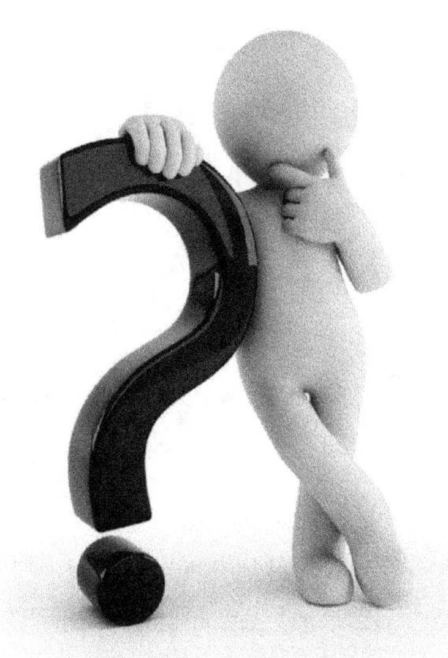

10. THE SUBSTANCE IS THE SYMPTOM

"This above all: To thine own self be true." —William Shakespeare

Before I discovered these principles, here's what I did: I binged on roast beef, bread and butter, goose liver pâté, ham, whole chickens, macaroni and cheese, croutons, non-dairy creamer with a spoon, whole sleeves of crackers, and of course, the ice cream-candy-cookie trilogy. This may sound disgusting (it disgusts me to remember), but it wasn't about the eating. The food was a symptom of a deeper challenge—being true to myself.

Until we get some self-honesty and seriously begin to look at ourselves, we may never move away from this unhealthy behavior. To focus on weight alone is to ignore the deeper issues. The substance (overeating) is the symptom, not the problem.

Focusing on weight alone is to ignore the deeper issues.

Our trouble usually begins with something unpleasant—an event or series of them—in our past, which causes us to react. In your past, there could have been a verbally abusive parent, a neglectful parent, sexual abuse—or any other traumatic experience, emotionally or physically.

People respond differently to stress from their pasts. Many overeat regularly, completely unaware of where the problem originated. Your unhealthy habit may stem from old messages playing in your head.

In fact, this is true of all our harmful patterns. Usually there is an unrelated cause, but our response was to eat too much every day. The excess weight was the result.

WEED THE GARDEN

In Romans 7:15, the Apostle Paul says, "*I do not understand what I do. For what I want to do I do not do, but what I hate I do.*"

Can you relate to Paul's words? If so, why do you do this? Is it a question of self-neglect, or is something deeper going on?

This is the time to sit down, journal, and learn about yourself. These "old messages" in your head have the potential to control you today. It's time to weed the garden. Identify your undesirable behavior and its causes. Dig deep into your past and your life and find those bitter roots. Once you pull them up and directly face the facts, the weeds will be gone forever.

St. Paul also wrote in Hebrews 12:15, "*See to it that no one misses the grace of God and that no bitter root grows up to cause trouble and defile many.*"

In other words, your actions may seem to only affect you, but in reality, your behavior can affect a whole family or community of people.

So don't fool yourself by saying you are the only one who suffers from your deeds.

IF THE SUBSTANCE IS THE SYMPTOM, THEN WHAT'S THE PROBLEM?

Here's where the hard part comes. This may require getting up earlier each morning to journal or meditate. You may have to wait for the answers, but while you wait, start applying the principles in this book.

The famous quote by Aristotle applies here, "The whole is greater than the sum of its parts." If you attack the issues from different angles, you will reap rewards that far surpass your efforts. Your results will be synergistic.

For example, you can begin to clean out unnecessary food in your kitchen and pantry over the next few weeks. You can begin a short, five-minute meditation each morning. In the afternoon, you might walk a few blocks for exercise. These little actions don't require much time. The interaction of these small steps will have a positive effect on your perspective. Momentum will build, and you will desire more of this energy. Why? Because it feels good!

HOMEWORK

Identify something that bothers you regularly and causes you to eat too much. The food may not be the real problem, but instead may be a symptom. Only when the basic cause is addressed, will the symptom finally go away.

Can you identify at least one thing in your life you feel is directly related to how you eat? When did the overeating begin? Did something happen—an accident, a horrific event? Or was it a relationship with a sibling, parent, relative—or someone else?

Record your findings in your journal. Is there someone you think about who needs your forgiveness? Are you still angry about something that happened years ago? Even if they were at fault and you were the victim, they still need to be forgiven in order for you to be free of destructive eating.

Are you stuffing down negative emotions by eating? Can you express yourself another way? Do you have a friend or counselor with whom you can confide?

Once you are able to forgive, you will let go of these toxic feelings. You will realize your overeating played a part in your lack of forgiveness. When you finally let go and forgive, the need for excess food will evaporate.

If you have come this far, you can congratulate yourself. You have taken a huge step forward. This is the beginning of your new life.

FOUR COMMON PROBLEMS OF OVEREATERS

Listed below are examples of problems overeaters may experience. This list may help you determine some inner tensions you need to address.

1. Being overwhelmed by feelings is a common reason why many people overeat. Feelings can manifest themselves in many ways, so I will mention only a few of them here. The reasons for emotional eating are as varied as the number of individuals, so I may not list all that apply to you.

Here are some ways people have eaten to suppress their emotions. I'm sure you can add some to this list:

- We hated our job (feelings of obligation or pressure)
- We were always stressed for time, so we ate too fast (pressure to over-accomplish)
- We experienced traffic frustration
- We had a confrontation during the day that stressed us out

(irritation)

- We did poorly on a test (anger)
- We did really well on a test (excitement)
- We were relieved at finishing a project, a semester at school, or graduating (relief)
- We got fearful about money
- Our income suddenly increased (excitement)
- We lost a large sum of money (depression, fear)
- We avoided an uncomfortable situation (fear)
- We didn't want to involve ourselves in an uncomfortable relationship (fear)
- We didn't want to set goals out of fear of failure
- We avoided making a decision (fear)
- We had negative self-talk, such as, "I'll always be fat", "this binge won't make a difference; I'll start dieting tomorrow", or "I'll never be able to lose weight."
- We fell in love or out of love (excitement or depression)
- We got unexpected news, such as divorce, a firing or medical news (any negative emotions)
- We got a ticket for a traffic violation (anger)
- We felt sorry for ourselves (self-pity)
- We came home from work and needed to decompress and there was the food in our face, accessible and immediate (stress relief).

Everybody is, at some time, overwhelmed by feelings. Your homework is to identify these times and to learn when you have less self-control. Your self-discovery and your formula will consist of gaining awareness of these characteristics, and working with them to overcome them. Once you identify them, you can begin the process of healing by addressing those needs in healthy and effective ways instead of compensating for them with food.

2. Failure to establish and enforce one's boundaries can get people into a lot of trouble. This is as true in any area of life as it is with food, but we emotional eaters usually head to food as a solution first. Boundaries can be food-specific, such as "I can't sample anymore at the grocery store—it gets out of hand and I eat too much." On the other hand, boundaries don't have to be directly related to food, such as, "I can't date this woman anymore. She's negative, and I feel bad when I'm around her".

3. Isolation seems to be a common syndrome among problem overeaters. Often, the unhealthy eating is done in secret, since we know our behavior is wrong and we are ashamed. If we can force ourselves to reach out to others instead, the food may no longer be necessary to cope with painful aspects of life. We will be using healthier, more effective alternatives. In other words, we share our burdens.

Please don't confuse secret eating with "down time" or the need to occasionally pull back and take time for ourselves. This is a healthy endeavor, and it is up to us to determine what our needs are in this area. However, isolating is unhealthy for those of us who tend to overeat, and may be difficult to change if we are entrenched in the habit. Withdrawal from others is also common for those who suffer from depression.

How do you determine your needs for solitude? Consider these questions.

- Is your calendar booked solid each day, with no empty space?
- Are you on a treadmill of busyness, and don't know how to get off?
- Are you irritable, angry, or cry easily, and don't know why?
- When you arise in the morning, do you dread your busy days?

- What's going on with your relationship to God? Did you used to have a daily quiet time and then stop?

A "yes" answer to one or more questions will indicate you aren't taking enough time for yourself. Think about something that you can change today to promote inner peace. You can resume your devotions, engage in more activities you enjoy, journal about your feelings, and allow more white space in your calendar days.

A habit takes twenty-one days to take "root" in an individual. If you realize isolated eating may be a problem, why not connect with friends instead?

For example, instead of going home right after work and opening the refrigerator, why not meet someone for some good conversation for an hour? Do this for the next three weeks, and you will have changed your life.

4. Our need to rejuvenate is a spiritual function that parallels a physical one. We can restore ourselves physically via sleep and rest, but what exactly does this mean in a spiritual sense? Here again, you will have to work your formula to determine your own needs.

People's requirements for spiritual refreshment differ tremendously. Some feel they need a certain amount each day. Others don't feel a need for spiritual things, yet don't recognize their vacuum. This lack of recognition causes problems for them.

When you start the process of self-discovery, your need for time alone may increase. That's not such a bad thing either, because when you understand yourself better, your self-care will increase. Doing things you know are right for you will become easier as you focus on your deepest needs and find your path to real rejuvenation. You will develop your ability to listen to your heart. You will have more of a desire to be alone in stillness and silence.

So how do you do this? Let's start by looking at two different types of individuals—the introvert and the extrovert. Read the following stories and determine with which you most closely identify.

JAN'S STORY

Jan was basically introverted. She liked being alone, and yet she was ashamed of it, because she thought she was different. She neglected to make extra time to putter in her house and do things that seemed unimportant, even though she needed these things to refresh her spirit.

She always had her earphones in her ears, the TV going, the radio going in her car and activities planned for every moment of every day. She was overweight and miserable, but she was also open-minded to new ideas. When she slowly allowed herself to accept her need to rejuvenate, she found she really liked meeting her needs in this area.

She eventually lost her shame and was no longer afraid to say to someone that she needed time alone. The weight began to come off because she was feeding her emotional hunger by taking better care of herself instead of eating.

Introverts recharge their batteries by getting quiet time away from others. Even if they are in the public eye—politicians, actors, and others—their introverted nature needs alone-time to decompress.

PATRICK'S STORY

Patrick was an extrovert and knew it. He had a strong sense of self and didn't deny his need for mingling among others and attending social events. However, he had a problem. His wife was an introvert who resented Patrick's always inviting people over to their house, interrupting her downtime. She felt violated and hurt every time he brought a guest into their space.

Unfortunately, their marriage didn't survive this obstacle, and they eventually divorced. The divorce might have been prevented if both spouses understood each other's needs for rejuvenation and developed a compromise.

Extroverts recharge their batteries by socializing and mingling among others. They may work in isolation—musical composers, authors, and others—but they have an inborn need for socialization.

Regardless of whether you are an introvert or an extrovert, both types need quiet time each day for introspection and spiritual development. Like the color of your eyes, you are primarily introverted or extroverted at birth. This is something you can't change. Therefore, it is good for you to understand your basic nature and to embrace the practices that feed your soul.

Finding your need for downtime is at the heart of your process of self-discovery. From this will stem all sorts of revelations. This is the foundation for a healthy lifestyle and permanent weight loss.

HOMEWORK

Look at some specific areas with food that you continue to be unsuccessful at. For example, suppose you lose control and overeat when you come home from the office after a hard day.

Try setting just one boundary and keeping it for a few weeks. In this case, you could try eating a prepared snack on the way home from work and immediately going for a walk when you arrive home. Continue this action at least three weeks, until this becomes a habit. You are setting a new boundary for yourself, one that gives you the space to unwind in a different way than overeating. When you become successful at this one change, you will actually enjoy the new habit. Then you can begin to move forward.

Following are some boundaries my clients have established for themselves:

- Planning their meals in advance, or at least having quick and healthy things to grab at all times

- Honoring their need for quiet time so they can be productive when it matters

- Not worrying about what others think of them and getting away from people-pleasing

- Communicating to one's spouse (in a loving way) that they need space tonight and want to be left alone.

Determine your individual boundaries and stick to them. This is vital to any success in life. Call them what you will—limitations, parameters, personal needs—all are paths to healthy change. If you regard them as negative or stifling, you may feel an inner resistance to change. Surprisingly, setting these boundaries will give you more freedom to be yourself!

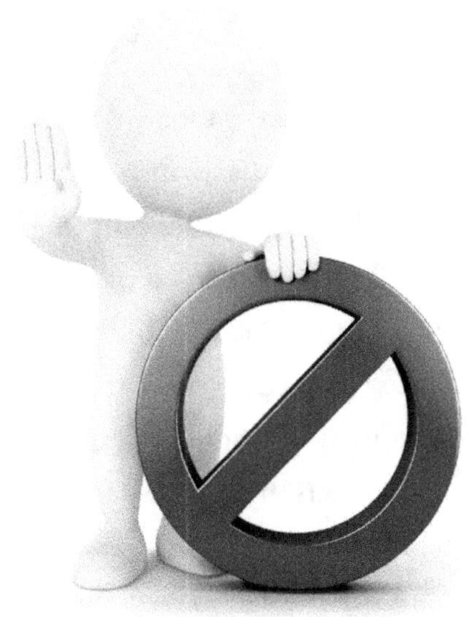

11. SUGAR: HOW SWEET IT ISN'T

"Be not deceived by the first appearance of things, for show is not substance."
—English Proverb

Sugar! Candy, cookies, cakes, ice cream, milk shakes, sweet treats, bonbons, chocolate, and more chocolate galore! Visions of a colorful, childlike, confection-laden, Willy Wonka's Chocolate Factory[vi] world dominates our thoughts during a crisis (or any other convenient time, for that matter).

America, we have a problem. We are so busy getting things done, working to achieve, saving for retirement, and taking care of business we have neglected our bodies way too long. We forget if we don't have a healthy body, we won't be able to accomplish much. Then, at the first sign of stress, we run toward sugary stuff for comfort, as if that's the appropriate response for each and every conflict. So, what happens is we develop another problem on top of the original issue. Life becomes even more complex.

We eat to our heart's desire. Whatever we want, whenever we feel like it, and however we choose, we do not deny ourselves—except, of course, that first week of January. Our intentions are good, but the motivation doesn't last. We fall back into our old patterns of stress eating, over-indulging, and maybe even bingeing. We must have our "poison." We indulge, and we are ashamed of ourselves.

Many of us have become wiser about the ways we neglect our health. Even if we realize we need to do better, often we can't. We find so much conflicting information, enough to make our heads spin. How do we weed through the garden of sly sales tactics to reach the flower of truth? We simply don't have time to figure it all out. Therefore, we continue on the unhappy road we've paved for ourselves and fear poor health in our future.

This section covers several areas pertaining to sugar. The first will focus on what a sugar gram is, e.g., how many grams per day would be considered in the healthy range.

The second part addresses the nutrition label. How do you know the quantity you are consuming? Is there an easy way to visualize that? We know where to find the sugar grams on the label, but how do we convert that into something we can relate to?

The third part addresses the deceptive labeling practices of manufacturers to allure us into buying their product. There's an easy way to know if a product has sugar in it, despite what the label says.

THE SUGAR GRAM

What exactly is a sugar gram? Well, like most of us know, a gram is a metric unit of weight. Although it's pretty small, this is the measure listed on a nutrition label.

How many grams per day are considered in the healthy range? According to the American Heart Association, up to 37.5 grams per day for men and about 25 grams per day for women are within a healthy range.

THE NUTRITION LABEL

Grams on a nutrition label can be a confusing quantity to understand. It's hard to know how much sugar we are actually consuming. To help visualize this, take the total grams in each serving and divide that number by 4. The following example uses a regular (non-diet), 12-ounce cola:

Serving Size 1 can (12 fl oz)
Serving Per Container 1

Amount Per Serving	
Calories 140	
	% Daily Values*
Total Fat 0g	**0%**
Saturated Fat 0g	**0%**
Trans Fat 0g	
Cholesterol 0mg	**0%**
Sodium 45mg	**2%**
Total Carbohydrate 39g	**13%**
Dietary Fiber 0g	**0%**
Sugars 39g	
Protein 0g	**0%**

How strange it is that the serving size is in ounces (English unit of measure), yet the amount of sugar per serving is in grams (metric). Can this be more obscure? Most of us don't take the trouble to determine how much they consume. But since it's important to us, let's figure this out the easy way.

Most restaurants don't serve sugar cubes anymore, but do you recall what one looks like? If not, then you do know what a packet of sugar looks like. They are both 4 grams of sugar, or one teaspoon. Look at these pictures.

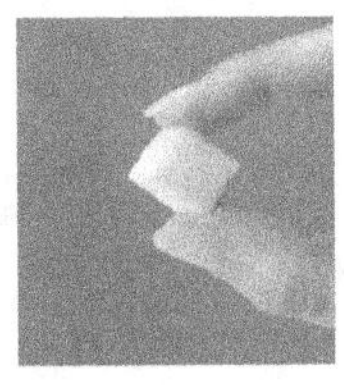
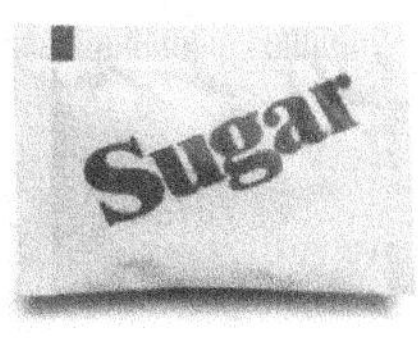

A packet of sugar is usually 4 grams or 1 teaspoon of sugar. So, considering the nutrition label of the 12-ounce cola, do you see the sugars listed are 39 grams?

39 Grams ÷ 4 Grams ~ 10

That is, 10 teaspoons, 10 sugar cubes, or 10 packets of sugar. This is a new perspective, isn't it? Did you realize you were consuming that much sugar in a 12-ounce non-diet soda?

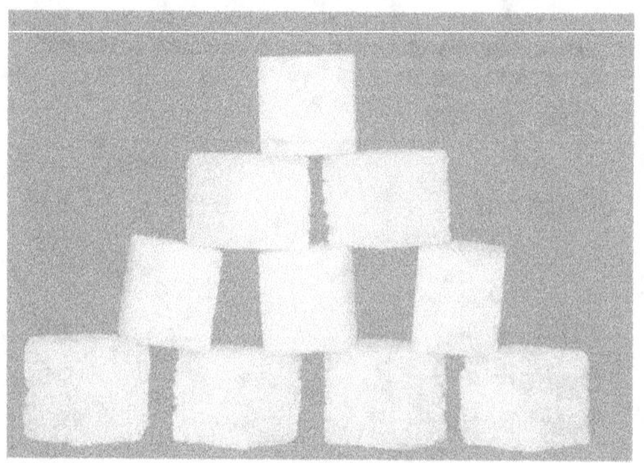

HOMEWORK

Begin today at your home. For each item you eat, look at the grams of sugar on the nutrition label. Then, divide the sugar grams by 4. Take the American Heart Association's recommendation of staying under 37.5 grams of sugar for men (a little more than 9 sugar cubes, sugar packets, or teaspoons) and 25 grams of sugar for women (a little more than 6). This activity will give you a starting point to measure your progress toward a diet lower in sugar. Your body will thank you!

DECEPTIVE LABELING PRACTICES

You probably know the primary motive of food manufacturers is to sell products. But do you realize they don't care one iota about your health?

Okay, perhaps that is more of a probability. This final section might be the most revealing, so get ready.

SUGAR IN THE LISTS OF INGREDIENTS

Once upon a time, a consumer could read the ingredients to find sugar content. If it was the first ingredient, then the majority of that product would consist of sugar.

Food manufacturers caught on to consumer's dislike of sugar years ago, so they have learned how to conceal the content by using different names for sugar in the ingredients list. Here are just a few of the names these manufacturers use to conceal the truth: barley malt, cane juice crystals, fruit juice concentrate, sorbitol, and maltodextrin.[vii]

To really know the sugar content, you must now look at the total grams of sugar on the nutrition label itself, not simply the ingredient list.

CLEVER LABELING FOR "SUGAR-FREE"

Here is the FDA's definition of "sugar free:"

> "Defined in Title 21 of the Code of Federal Regulations 101.60(c) (21 CFR 101.60(c)) as a claim that may be used on a food that contains less than 0.5 g of sugars, as defined in § 101.9(c)(6)(ii), per reference amount customarily consumed and per labeled serving (21 CFR 101.60 (c))."

What does "less than 0.5 g" and "per reference amount customarily consumed and per labeled serving" mean? How can these be manipulated on the food labels?

The FDA says in order for a food to be considered sugar-free, it has to consist of less than one-half of a gram of sugar per serving. That's pretty straightforward, even though the wording is a little—*uh*—wordy. What actually happens is the manufacturers know consumers will be attracted to "Sugar Free" on a label. They make the serving size small enough to fit into the FDA'S parameter. They are now legally able to call their product "sugar-free."

Your best bet is to notice the serving size. Multiply the grams per serving (on the nutrition label) by the number of servings you consume. Then, to visualize the number of sugar packets that quantifies, divide the grams by four. That's how much sugar you are eating.

> **Multiply the grams per serving by the number of servings you consume. That's how much sugar you are eating.**

SUGAR SEDUCTION

Even after my weight loss, I struggled with the sugar for many years. I didn't want to give it up. There was some kind of emotional connection there: I associated sweet foods with comfort, love, and fun. Frosting, candy, pastries, cookies, and cakes are pretty and colorful. When I ate, I was reminded of a time with no worries or responsibilities.

Indulging in sweet treats was an attempt to recapture these feelings, like an escape. Even into my forties, I would experience only a few brief spells of being sugar-free. During these times, I felt fantastic. I knew it was because I was taking care of my body and doing what I truly needed to do to feel good mentally and physically. Productivity and contentment increased, and I accomplished much with renewed courage and determination. Plus, I had more energy!

Then, I experienced phases where I succumbed to the desire once again—not so much a physical desire, because there was no craving due to my being abstinent for an extended time. This was an emotional desire, one for a different life, a longing for fun, and good times. I sought happiness from the sweets, but they could never deliver.

Deep down, I knew the sugar wouldn't provide me with inner peace. But I went there anyway, knowing what the consequences would be. Once I relented, I wanted some every night without exception. I couldn't resist it. The cravings got worse, the amounts I consumed increased, and sometimes I would even get ill from eating so much. Hangovers greeted me in the mornings, similar to that of an alcoholic.

Being disgusted with myself was an understatement. The weight crept up. More time was spent in the gym, compensating for the indulgences. Eventually, motivation overcame me, and I stopped eating sugar, cold turkey, resulting in physical withdrawal. My body was uncomfortable, and I was depressed for several days.

Then I felt better and stayed sugar-free for another phase, only to start again at some point. This craziness went on for decades, going back and forth from being sugar-free to sugar-full, not unlike a yo-yo dieter. Even a small amount could trigger the cravings. I became insatiable and wanted more and more. I never got to the place where I was satisfied with a small amount. The more I ate the more I wanted. The longer this went on, the emptier I felt.

This life was a distraction from my goals. What I really wanted to do was to meet all types of people, explore different career endeavors, and try new activities. So long as I was doing the yo-yo thing with sugar, I remained in a state of paralysis. I lost confidence in myself and had no self-esteem. This mindset prevented me from reaching for my true desires.

It's almost as if two people warred inside me: a good person and a bad person. At this point, the bad person seemed to be winning the battle.

Do you relate to my story? Sugar is many people's most common trigger food. Here's what you can do when you find yourself craving sugar and don't want to give in:

- Recognize that sugar is a problem for you. Open your mind to new choices to change your behavior and/or environment.
- Take a moment to acknowledge the agitation driving you to eat.

Sometimes simply getting in touch with your feelings takes away the craving for a sugar escape.

- Don't try to substitute any other food for the craving, because that would likely make the craving more powerful.

- If you must consume something, make a cup of hot tea without sweetener. The warmth is soothing and works wonders to carry your body through that craving. Leave the kitchen, and sit in a quiet spot to sip your tea. I promise: it works every time!

- Divert your focus to something productive. Help someone else.

- Remember—this too shall pass.

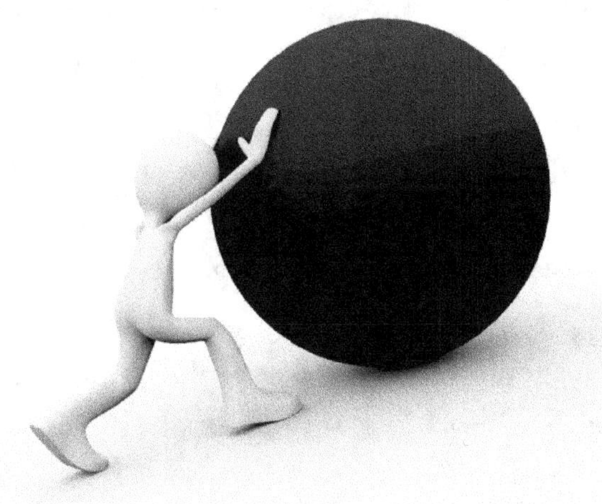

12. DETERMINATION AND DEPENDENCY

"Pride goes before destruction, a haughty spirit before a fall."
—Proverbs 16:18

Have you ever worked so hard and so long to achieve something, only to meet with discouragement and failure? Do you wonder if you are ineffective, spinning your wheels, and wasting your time? Why not just give up and accept yourself as a fat person who was never meant to be thin? Do you ever ask, "What does it take to be thin?" Has giving up become a realistic option?

CHEF: If this is you, do you see that you might be making progress with these thoughts?

You: *How can this be? How can I possibly be on the right track when I'm about to give up on the whole thing?*

CHEF: Aha!

You: *Oh no, not this again!*

CHEF: No, really! Ask yourself this question: what would it feel like to release your burden and draw closer to God in your hunger? He wants a relationship with you. Could it be He is using your struggle with food and weight to get your attention?

Like most people, I want to do things alone and take pride in my results. I want to be able to say, "Yes, I did that on my own." However, the longer I tried to lose the weight and gain control by myself, the more I failed.

All I'm suggesting is that you take this same mental approach to achieve permanent weight loss. If you do, your success will be a result of your efforts along with God's power.

So keep this idea in your mind when you start having small victories, and always give God the credit.

With a different mindset than before, your success will be a result of your efforts alongside God's power. Keep this idea in your mind. When you succeed in the smallest victory, give God the credit.

TAPPING INTO HIS POWER

What are some prayers or affirmations you like? When you are feeling the need to resist overeating, you can call on the Lord. Use His power. Some examples are:

- I always eat just what my body needs, and not one bite more.
- I am making progress every day.
- I take care of my temple, and I treat it with respect.

BIBLE VERSES THAT MAY HELP

"For we are God's fellow workers; you are God's field, God's building."
—1 Corinthians 3:9
"What, then, shall we say in response to this? If God is for us, who can be against us?" —Romans 8:31
"I can do everything through him who gives me strength." —Philippians 4:13

WRITE

Finally, if you get obsessive thoughts about food—or anything, for that matter—write. If you get upset during a conversation with a friend—write. If you have a disagreement with your spouse—write. If you are feeling happy—write. If you are feeling depressed—write. Do you get the picture? I hope so!

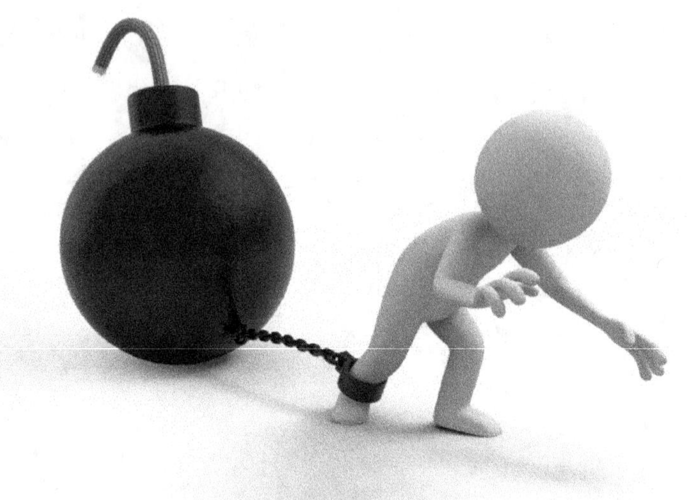

13. TRIGGERS

"A life of reaction is a life of slavery, intellectually and spiritually. One must fight for a life of action, not reaction."—Rita Mae Brown

A trigger is anything that has a negative influence on your ability to control your eating. It doesn't have to be a food, or it could even be healthy fare. Here are four types:

- Substance
- Situational
- Behavioral
- Circumstantial

SUBSTANCE TRIGGERS

When you eat certain items, do you have a difficult time stopping, or do you eat until you finish the whole package? If so, you may have a craving problem. To make matters worse, the more those items are eaten, the stronger the craving will be the next day, at the same time, for the same thing. It's a vicious cycle, extremely difficult to escape.

Junk and empty calories are high on the list: bread and butter, an open bag or bowl of anything sitting on the counter, saying, "I'm available, so come eat me!" Others are cookies, candy, pastries, "finger foods" (chips, crackers, and nuts). I could go on, but you probably get the picture by now and already have thought of a couple yourself. If you can't handle having something in your house, don't buy it. If someone else brought it in, you can ask him or her to hide it so you won't find it.

It's hard for anyone to overcome these cravings, and cold turkey withdrawal can be very uncomfortable. If you are trying to rid yourself of sugar, for example, try to offset that compulsion by having a low-carbohydrate, high-protein meal before you eat the sugar. You can also eat something high in protein with it, like nuts on top of frozen yogurt. But only do this after eating a healthy dinner. If this experiment doesn't work, it may be time to eliminate these items from your diet. This approach may be the best solution for you.

Suppose you say, "Well, I'll finish this up, and then I won't get it again at the store." I promise, it will take you that much longer to reach your goals, because you're procrastinating on beginning the process. What's more, every time you go to the grocery store, you'll be torn about what you should buy. Although you know you need to lose weight, you haven't really decided changing your lifestyle is a priority. Yet your conscience tells you this is what you need to do, hence the conflict.

GUILTY CONSCIENCE?

If you feel guilty throwing out food—even if it's bad for you ("it's wasteful!" or "think of all those starving people on the other side of the world!"), try doing one of several things:

- **Put it in a big bowl** outside to feed the stray animals.

- **Toss it** in the trash bin and dump the kitty litter on it—or some other undesirable mess that would make it inedible.

- **Get your significant other** (or trusty friend) to throw it out for you (and hide it so you won't find it!).
- **Flush it** down the toilet. (Don't tell your plumber I said that.)
- **Give it away**.

NON-FOOD RELATED TRIGGERS

Sometimes things unrelated to food prompt us to eat. In order to lose weight, we need to focus on and deal with these exact things. As long as we deny these problems, we will remain incapable of resolving our weight issue.

SITUATIONAL TRIGGERS

Can you think of recurring difficulties that set off an impulse to overeat or binge? For example, a situational trigger can be work-related, such as a regular meeting that causes stress. It could be the periodic hiring or firing of an employee, or even a particular catered event. Another such situation could be going to a party and "socializing" right by the food table, making it an easy temptation to indulge in too much food.

Do you identify with any of these scenarios? Can you think of one with which you regularly struggle? How does it manifest in your life? What usually happens when you face it? Unless you are aware of what's happening, you will automatically fall into the pattern of overeating in these cases.

Please note that situational triggers don't have to be negative to spark overindulging. Yearly family get-togethers, joyful holiday festivities, and summer vacations can also be situational triggers.

The keys to recognizing your situational triggers are "periodic" or "regularly occurring."

BEHAVORIAL TRIGGERS

These are catalysts that cause and encourage *unconscious* eating. Do you enjoy eating while you're engaged in a specific kind of activity? If so, you may eat and eat, but don't realize how much you've consumed. Do you get lost in thought on the computer or in a book? Is this an escape for you? Does the eating calm your spirit?

If you identify with this trigger, please write about why you do it. Is there a healthier, more effective way you can nurture yourself? How about a long hot bath with essential oils, meditation, a nap, or a bike ride?

Trigger behaviors can include eating a bag of chips in front of the TV, or eating at the computer while you work. These types of triggers are often done in isolation. If you engage in this type of eating, do you plan to have time alone in order to do this?

Do you admit you *want* to engage in unconscious eating from time to time? Try to think about the consequence of the weight piling on and how powerless you feel about the whole situation.

If you engage in behavioral triggers, you have two choices:

- **Continue on** the way you have been going. Gain weight and stay in denial of the problem. Convince yourself you like to be fat, you've always been fat, and will forever be fat. I can't tell you how many times I've heard people say, "My mom was fat, her mom was fat, and I'm fat. I guess that's just the way I am." Do you say this? If so, why? Is it an excuse, or a cop-out from taking action to improve your life? Is it laziness?

- **Change the behavior** in some way. You can cut back, you can change the food or the activity, or you can stop doing them together. However, if one attempts to stop the food, and continue the activity, there will be a void. There will still be that urge to eat while engaging in the activity. Something—some action or behavior—will have to replace the food.

If you choose the second option, in the case of television, simply turning off the TV might do the trick. But in the case of computer work (probably a necessary thing), something will have to be substituted. In this case, keep a large glass of water right next to your computer. You might also try brewing a cup of hot tea to sip on while you work. You can also try rearranging the furniture, adding candles, or changing the ambiance in different ways. Regardless of what you change, you will notice that something is different at first, and there will be some discomfort. Move through these feelings, and know it will get easier.

Finally, you can try calling someone before you sit down. Tell them you want to work without eating. Ask your friend to hold you accountable. Ask them to call you later, at a specific time, to check on you. Do this every time you sit at the desk until the cravings no longer torment you and you have regained control.

CIRCUMSTANTIAL TRIGGERS

Everyone has unexpected things that happen at the most inconvenient times. An unexpected project gets dumped on you at work, car repairs, the death of a pet, and sudden home maintenance costs are just a few of the burdens I've faced at one time or another.

How do you react to these circumstances? Do they trip an eating response in you? Circumstantial triggers can cause overeating of any type of food, leading to a portion-control problem. This dilemma is a behavioral issue rather than a substance one—or, it can be both, depending on what is consumed. In any case, if you are prone to reacting to life's "bumps in the road" by overeating, then what you really need to do is recognize your emotion preceding the first bite and then deal with the situation differently.

HOMEWORK

Take a moment to list in your journal at least two examples of each: food triggers, trigger situations, trigger behaviors, and circumstantial triggers. Your examples will become red flags for you to recognize so you can avoid getting into trouble with the food. They will ultimately help you reach your goals.

Do most, if not all of those foods on your list contain either sugar, white flour, or both? There may be a rogue here or there: caffeine has been a trigger for some. But mostly, the culprits are processed, sweet, salty, crunchy items. If you relate to this, then you can bet anything with significant amounts of these ingredients will cause a reaction in you.

Later in the book, you will have an opportunity to make your grocery list. At that time, you will become more aware of what's in the products you buy. You will then be able to avoid foods that are high in ingredients that disagree with you.

When you consider your triggers, don't underestimate their "pull" to get you off-track. You must be honest with yourself if you plan to eliminate the right things from your kitchen. You will need to change your behaviors and choose to respond differently to life's ups and downs. All of your positive actions will hone and improve your formula.

CONFESSIONS OF A CLOSET-EATER

Readers beware! Here is a list of some of the ways people have behaved with regard to food. The list is not exhaustive, and I'm sure other closet eaters can add to it. Read it and laugh! But mostly, be determined that you will never:

- Bury food wrappers in the trash so no one will find them to see what has been eaten.

- Hide in the closet or bathroom in order to eat secretly.

- Lying to someone that we didn't eat something when in actuality, we gorged on it.

- Eat leftovers from the guest's plates after clearing the table.

- Lie to others and ourselves about our physical hunger.

- Deny to others and ourselves about how much we had eaten.

- Fast for several days to lose weight for an event, then after the event, bingeing on candy to break the fast.

- Run the disposal while regurgitating the binge so the person in the other room wouldn't hear.

- Wake up at 3:00 a.m. to grocery shop at a 24-hour store in order to binge in private upon our returning home.

- Purchase bags of groceries for the sole purpose of bingeing on the contents.

- Hit all the grocery stores for the specials on sugary cereal, cake mix, ice cream, cookies, candy, icing and anything else to binge on.

- Be so possessive over "your" food at home that you label to protect it from being eaten by someone else.

- Get resentful when someone eats it.

- Dig someone else's leftover food out of the trash, dusting the ants off and eating it.

- Tell the grocery store cashier you're buying a super-large cake for an office party, then proceed to go home and binge on the whole thing.

Those of us who have overcome this kind of unhealthy behavior can laugh at ourselves today. Thank God, we're not there anymore! I hope you never will be, but if you are, know you can overcome these awful habits. This should also give you more incentive to engage in self-discovery, knowing that others have preceded you.

Self-examination is the key to the door that will open a world of new ideas, so if you didn't work some of the homework assignments or questions earlier in the book, go back and complete them now. If you took a half-hearted approach on some, do them again. Perhaps you will learn more the second time around.

Self-examination is the key to the door that will open a world of new ideas.

Whatever you do, never stop working! Let this book be the beginning of a life of introspection. Look for further ways to deepen your relationship with your inner self. Weight loss and maintenance are just around the corner and will be by-products of your efforts.

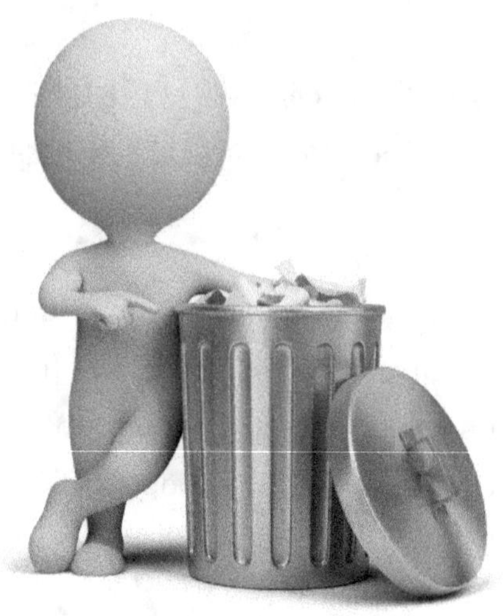

14. DUMP THE JUNK!

"We must be willing to get rid of the life we've planned, so as to have the life that is waiting for us. The old skin has to be shed before the new one can come." —Joseph Campbell

God will give you a higher degree of self-control, if you truly seek it. You can achieve this through a combination of accurate basic nutritional knowledge and self-honesty (with that last one being the biggest part).

Once you see your progress, your desires will change. You will want to eat nutrient-dense foods. You will no longer want the empty calories. Your yearnings for good health will destroy the craving for junk!

When you work these principles, you'll develop intuition, which will further enable you to improve. Are you ready to become the best person you can be? It starts with you, right now. Here are some promises:

- You will experience a new relationship with food. You will begin to listen to your body.

- You will have the power to abstain from excess food when your body has had enough.

- You will develop that wonderful quality called honesty.

- You will learn to read your body's hunger and satiety signals.

- You will avoid negative situations by staying away from self-sabotaging thoughts, people, and places. This knowledge will help you make the right decisions along the way if you accept your temptations, limitations, or vulnerabilities.

- You will remain vigilant about your boundaries, and then protect yourselves from falling back into old patterns of eating.

- No food tastes better than the reward of healthy living.

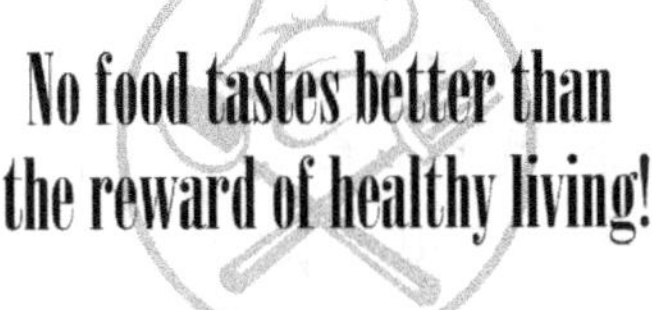

CAN YOU FIX YOUR BROKEN BAROMETER?

Have you abused food so intensely for so many years that you wonder if you can ever be restored to a normal lifestyle?

Stop right here. What's "normal?" Does it mean how someone else eats and behaves? Or is it an ideal you have in your mind as to what you are supposed to be like?

The only program that will be successful for you is one you formulate around your individuality. The quickest way to fail is to look at what someone else is doing and try to make that happen in your life exactly as it appears to you. Now, you *can* take ideas from others you admire and incorporate them into your life, one at a time. This way, you tailor each facet to the new "you." But an outright attempt to immediately transform yourself into another person can only be met with failure.

Developing your own formula takes time and effort. It's long and boring. The weight loss doesn't occur quickly, either. Furthermore, since your life and body change over time, you periodically need to recalibrate your formula. Simply put, we are living differently and have created a new awareness about ourselves. This mindset must be maintained if we are to remain successful.

One day, you will be able to distinguish between physical hunger, boredom, depression, or some other emotion masquerading as hunger. When you have a compulsion to eat, and you realize it's not a hunger-urge, you will take action to do something other than indulge. This is so empowering, and I know you look forward to having these victories again and again!

You will need to set boundaries that are food-related. An example would be to eat a small snack before you prepare dinner for your family. If you do this, you won't overeat during the preparation, 'tasting' as you cook. Another commitment could be social. For example, you could be more selective about which parties you attend, or with whom you associate. These changes are all your process of personalizing your formula. So stay in touch with your feelings, because they are the key to your success. They will guide you all the way.

When you learn to pay attention to your intuition, you will honor yourself. You will gain self-control over your eating choices, and your emotional barometer will stabilize. But this will occur only over time and with constant practice.

One day, you will be able to look back and see significant changes, including healthy adjustments to the foods you eat. You will also notice changes in the ways you respond to life in general. You are definitely going in the right direction!

Although you may have a certain weight in mind, you may never reach that ideal. However, as you keep following these principles, you will edge closer and closer to your goal.

SURPRISING RESULTS FROM WORKING YOUR FORMULA

Getting away from your formula for a time may be fun at first, but eventually becomes uncomfortable.

- You'll have strong urges to get back "on track" with your healthy eating plan.

- You'll look forward to aligning yourself to your formula more than being off it.

- You'll find yourself choosing a healthy lifestyle, instead of the bad choices you used to make.

- Because you have lost weight, others may suspect you are able to eat anything you want at any time.

- You'll find yourselves enjoying your formula—and your new life— more than ever.

- You'll try to convert others to find their own formula, knowing how much better they can feel.

Your weapon is your knowledge;
your ammunition is your faith;
and your success is within you!

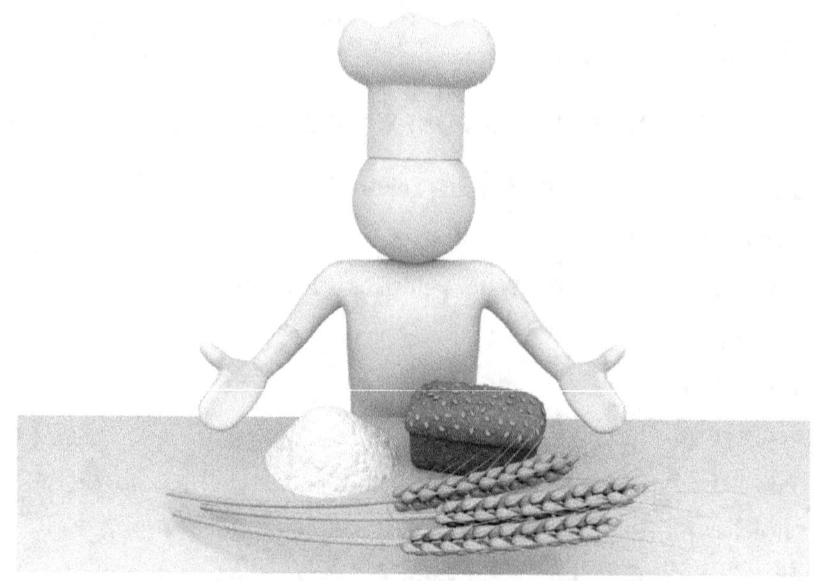

15. FALSE BREAD VS. THE TRUTH

"I am the bread of life. He who comes to me will never go hungry, and he who believes in me will never be thirsty." —John 6:35

Jesus is the Living Bread. He can be compared to whole, sprouted-grain bread that thoroughly nourishes the body's cells.

The false breads (gods) are like white bread, bleached to look pretty and perfect. They come with pretty and perfect packaging that promises so much. We are drawn to these alluring packages. Their grains are so milled they hardly need the body's digestion process. However, their grain is also stripped of all natural ingredients and nutrients, and then they are "enriched" with man's idea of the USRDA (United States Recommended Daily Allowance). It goes immediately into the bloodstream, bypassing all filters—no fiber to cleanse the intestines and no wheat germ for the body to slowly digest.

This false bread gives immediate satiety, denying the body what it was designed to do in the process of digestion. Over time, people may become addicted to it and even spit out the good whole-wheat bread because it tastes so foreign.

MY PERSPECTIVE

From the first time I put false philosophies in my system as a child, I tasted confusion. In fact, I grew up that way. I didn't know the Lord as a child, so I developed beliefs in fake truths. This "false bread" dwarfed my spiritual hunger, and I craved it more and more. I was full, yet I was hungry.

I learned to process life this way, looking for answers in the wrong places, expecting satisfaction from food, people, and things that were incapable of satisfying. I attempted to use others to satisfy a longing only Jesus can fill. The problem with processing life this way is I never found true contentment. I was constantly getting hurt—and then disappointed—by others. Where could I find satisfaction? I didn't know what I wanted, but I knew I hadn't found it. How would I get out of this pit?

Eventually, these conflicting messages became more acute than my hunger. I became obsessed with eating—when I could eat, whether or not I could be alone, how I could get my binge foods—and I was sucked into a lifestyle that consumed me so much I couldn't do anything else. This led me to question my previous philosophy, my source for my beliefs.

Over time, I was introduced to the True Bread. What I once spit out in disgust years before tasted new, nourishing, refreshing, and uplifting. It filled me in a miraculous way. There was no doubt in my mind this was the right path.

In spiritual things, there is One Truth, that of the Living God. There are other pseudo-truths that are manmade creations, manifested in different ways to appeal to the masses. In Matthew 7:13, Jesus says, "*Enter through the narrow gate.*" There are many ways man attempts to fill that soul-hole, but according to the Bible, there is only one way to fill it, and that is through the Son of God, Jesus Christ.

In spiritual things, there is One Truth, that of the Living God.

Something I ask my clients is, "Do you eat what you crave, or do you crave what you eat?" I let them think about it for a moment, and they usually respond with, "I don't know." I then suggest we can train our bodies to crave what we eat and *then* we will eat what we crave.

I didn't immediately crave a relationship with Jesus after opening my heart to Him. But I did know, somewhere deep inside of me, that He was the True Bread. I kept acting on this belief, and eventually came to crave the satisfaction He brought above all others. Only He can truly satisfy.

Draw close to Him, and He will draw close to you.

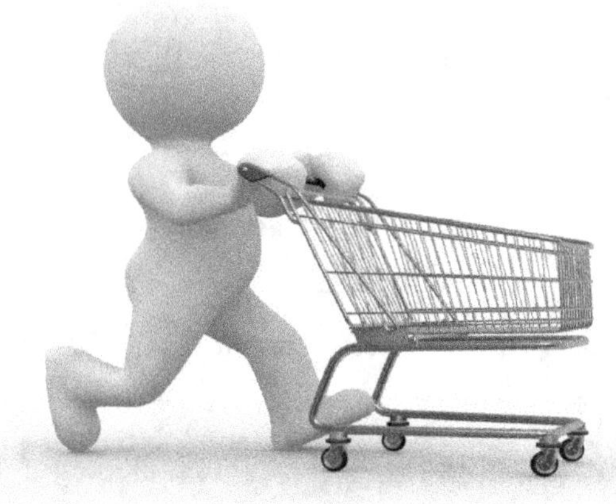

16. WALK THE AISLES AND READ BETWEEN THE LINES

Here's where the fun starts! Now you are ready to put a grocery list together based on the number of meals you expect to eat each day. You will be taken through a normal day in life and build your eating plan. This will be your most effective tool to crystallize your weight-loss goals and help you carry them out.

Which is more important: to eat less frequently or to eat fewer calories?

A recent study has determined that if you keep the calories the same, eating more frequent meals does not contribute to faster weight loss.[viii]

Cutting the number of calories to lose weight is the most effective way to achieve this. In addition, *how* we eat them contributes to satiety and more likely permanent weight loss.[ix] According to this study, if you want to produce permanent results, it takes both a caloric reduction plus more frequent meals.

Try this plan:

- Eat every few hours, instead of one big meal a day. You'll be less hungry and won't feel deprived.

- Choose foods that are less calorie-dense (low fat vs. high fat, for example) so you can eat a greater volume of food.

- Eat smaller portions to stay energized, not large servings that make you feel sluggish.

- Taper your meal size down toward the end of the day,[x] instead of having a small breakfast, average-sized lunch, and humongous dinner. You're going to bed soon after your evening meal. Why consume a bunch of calories you won't burn off? The time to eat a big meal (if ever) is early in the day. (I know, it's not fun that way. We seldom have company at breakfast.)

HOW MANY MEALS A DAY SHOULD I EAT?

I think we can all agree one huge meal a day is probably not the ideal way to lose weight.[xi] At the very best, you'd be physically uncomfortable, likely ranging from too full to too hungry (I'll share more on blood sugar levels later) or possibly mentally obsessed with the whole thing. At worst, losing the weight and permanently maintaining that loss would be hard to sustain with that kind of regimen if you were eating the same number of calories in that one meal as the total of the multiple meals of the day.

Right now, you might be eating only once per day. Others might be eating twice or three times. Let's just suppose you eat two times a day. My suggestion would be to increase by one meal each week until you reach a habit and frequency where you are satisfied between meals and don't feel you're hanging on until the next one.

Other indications you have reached this point are:

- You will gain a more positive outlook and be more excited about life in general.

- You will have an increase of mental energy to do the things you love doing.

- You will be more in tune with your body's hunger signs.

With this design, there will be no preoccupation with the program you've set for yourself, and you'll experience a freedom (maybe for the first time) from thinking about eating.

This is just the start. When you get results, you'll be so excited you will want more and be driven to work harder.

Your goal should be to find your ideal number of meals a day. Whatever your magic number is, press on. You'll find a comfort level with your lifestyle that's perfect for you.

With my current lifestyle, I find four to five meals a day is pretty comfortable. My program works for me right now, although it might change in the future. Keep this in mind: your personal formula will ebb and flow, but it's always in your control.

Increase your meal frequency with the mindset that you may or may not *maintain* that rate. This is the first step. The next task for you is to determine the quantity of food that goes on your grocery list, based on how many times you eat each day.

If you normally consume five to six meals a day, you will encounter situations when you eat more often (for example, if you travel and have gone through a time zone, or if you are burning the candle on both ends), or less (day-long meetings at work, long volunteer shifts, or involvement with something that makes you forget). Remember, you are only trying to arrive at an average plan.

How many meals per day are realistic for you? Consider your

calendar and lifestyle—not where you want to be, but where you are right now. How many are you willing to prepare each week? How much time do you have to invest in this? Is purchasing "ready-made," healthy foods an option for you? These can be expensive, but if you can afford them, they work great. Some companies even deliver to your door.

Where can you comfortably fit eating times in your schedule? In the example that follows, I'll illustrate a diet plan with three normal meals and several snacks spaced around them.

HOMEWORK

Calculate the number of meals you will try to consume each day and multiply that by seven. This will be the number of meals you'll be shopping for in your weekly trip.

Obviously, this is a guideline, and won't be a constant. There will be social activities, parties, trips out of town, and other events that take you away from eating at home. You may have some weeks in which you have purchased too much food. In any case, it's better to have extra on hand than not enough, because if you run out, this can sabotage your goals.

It's not a good feeling to find your stomach growling for food, facing an empty refrigerator and pantry. If you aren't completely honest with yourself, this might be an easy excuse to head for the grocery store or go out to eat.

There is a clear difference between making a conscious choice to do something deliberately, versus allowing circumstances to control you.

Keep your eyes focused on your goals, and you will soon be looking at success.

CLEAN THE KITCHEN!

"Be great in act, as you have been in thought." —William Shakespeare

It's time to clean out the old and make room for the new. Get rid of the junk—or as much as possible. This will prepare you to make a healthy grocery list and reaffirm your determination to keep those tempting things out of your house.

If you have children, a spouse, or roommate who is not on your weight-loss journey, you might encounter resistance removing their stuff. Do they need to keep their stash in a separate space so you can't see it? Can you make food purchases less tempting to you, yet similarly satisfying to them?

If you are resolved to win the war against overeating, their special food in the house shouldn't discourage you. You'll be sure to find ways to bypass the temptations.

HOMEWORK

Make a quick list of seductive edibles in your house. Your goal is to rid yourself of these items. Ask other household members to hide, keep in their room/office, or not display their treats in open, general areas. Dispose of your sabotaging substances by giving them away, eating them and purposing not to buy them again, or tossing them in the trash.

Be brave and determined! Set these things aside and dispose of them.

- Your local food pantry will accept unopened unexpired packages if you don't want to throw them away.
- Bring them to social clubs or group meetings.
- Pass them on to a friend who loves that item.

This "junk" can be any non-nutritious food or drink, or any item that tempts you to overeat or crave. These may include processed fare, snacks, chips, soda, drive-thru menu items, cookies, candy, or other provisions.

MAKING YOUR LIST

After you have cleaned the rubbish from your kitchen, your next step is to make a grocery list. Start your list with the healthy food you like. If you are unsure about whether or not to keep buying certain items, you can still get them for now. As you move through your journey, you'll learn more and more. You'll become more equipped to make the best choices in the grocery store. If you know something isn't good for you, simply avoid buying it. Ask a supportive friend to accompany you to the store if you need help with willpower at first.

If you aren't ready to totally abstain from something, why not buy a little less this week? If there is one junky thing you feel you cannot do without, keep it for now, but at least get rid of some other things.

Warning—what you eat affects your physiology when you alter your nutrition. The more abrupt your changes, the more difficult it may be to adjust.[xii] Symptoms may include moodiness, stomach upsets, gastro-intestinal distress and bloating, to name a few. So don't try to go from start to finish in one grocery trip. This is a process. Be gentle with yourself. Give your body enough time to adapt.

In addition, if you change your eating habits too fast, you will have a hard time adhering to a new plan. You'll be physically uncomfortable, become frustrated, and give up, sliding back to your old, comfortable habits. Don't pressure yourself to sprint toward your goal. Give yourself a little more time to get used to the program, and you're much more apt to be successful.

Make one or two small changes a week, but hold on to those and build on top of them. Nutritional adjustments need to be taken slowly. If you backslide and your eating is worse one week than the previous week, don't worry about it. Simply start where you stand and move on from that point.

Regular trips to the grocery store aren't an option. Regardless of your lifestyle, you must always have healthy choices at home to prevent sabotage to your formula. Dovetail your lifestyle with your shopping frequency to determine how often you need to go. In doing so, you'll keep these healthy choices in your refrigerator, freezer, and pantry. Finally, make it a priority to shop certain days of the week, and stick to them. Consider this as building another good habit.

Focus on your shopping and cooking at the same time to prepare you for the week ahead. Purchase plastic airtight containers for taking food with you wherever you go. Use a variety of sizes to portion your meals. Plan to freeze some meals you prepare.

HOMEWORK

Plan your weeks' meals and make your list. Ensure you have enough containers to freeze meals.

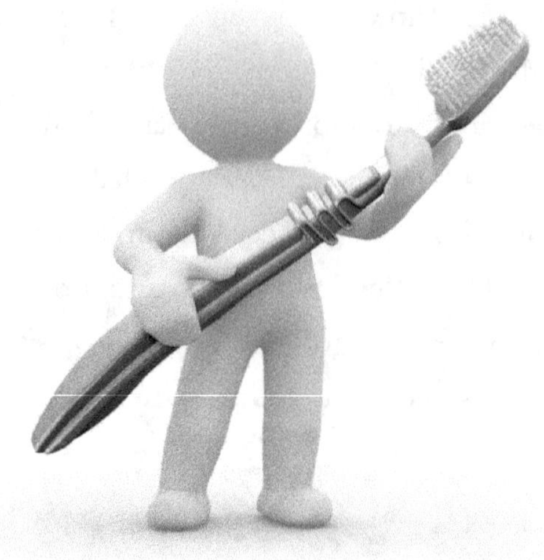

17. BRUSH YOUR TEETH!

"Character is simply habit long continued." —Plutarch

Eating healthfully should become such a part of your routine that you don't have to pay much attention to it. This can be a way of life for you, and you can learn to become emotionally detached from the process. You simply do it for the true goal: to sustain and prolong life with a lean and healthy body.

Here's a cute analogy regarding healthy nutritional habits. Do you remember the details of brushing your teeth? The color of the brush, brand of toothpaste, flavor, and how long you scrubbed this morning? Do you ever forget to do it? Rarely? How about flossing? Oh, I got some of you there!

If your dentist says to brush and floss your teeth daily, why wouldn't you? If you knew the best way to prevent gum disease was to do these tried-and-true daily practices, wouldn't you do them? Finally, if doing these things insures that your teeth remain in your skull, then it is to your advantage to do them regularly, right?

Brushing your teeth is something you do every day for your health—and details about it tend to get forgotten over time. In fact, after the initial taste of new toothpaste or impulse buy of that cool-looking toothbrush, it really doesn't matter if you have a certain flavor, brand, or color toothbrush. It's simply a part of your day you likely don't pay attention to.

Let's tie this analogy to your food and eating behavior. Do you remember all the details about every meal you ate yesterday? Perhaps. What about the day before? Maybe not so much. My point is that you might feel the food in front of you is the most important thing in your life, but when you gain perspective, it's really not!

Now, let's bring this closer to home. Most doctors recommend eating more veggies and fruits, and fewer sweets and red meats. This is good for you and actually helps prevent disease (stroke, heart disease, diabetes, etc). So, if you knew feeling super and energetic plus having the benefit of a stronger immune system were by-products of eating a healthy diet most days, then why not do it?

Eating is something we all do every day, and details tend to get forgotten. Taste and satisfaction lose importance as long as we have a healthy diet. After the initial bite, many of us may not even notice the rest of the meal.

You should eat in a non-negotiable fashion most of the time. Stop bargaining with yourself. Be your own parent and disciplinarian. You know what's best. If you do, you will begin *eating to live*, without any emotional attachment. You'll just do it, and it's done. But on the occasion when you do emphasize the food, whether it is a home-cooked, gourmet spread or a restaurant meal, enjoy it to the highest.

EMOTIONAL EATING

There is a world of difference between "eating to live" versus "living to eat." Not that you shouldn't enjoy your food. God created a variety of foods so we would enjoy eating. This is natural and healthy.

But do you insist on using your mother's recipes, dressing up every single meal, and ignore the fact that it's fattening and/or unhealthy? Do you have to prepare your food breaded or fried in order to be happy with your meal? If so, it's time to take the emotion out of the eating.

Most of the time, keep meal preparation simple and quick. I have news for you—food doesn't have to be the perfect gourmet experience to sustain life. Some meals can be a little boring, with steamed vegetables and low-fat meats. It's not a big deal to have a boring breakfast, lunch, or dinner. Just do it and move on with your life. Then, when you do spend more time preparing, you will savor your food as a planned diversion from your normal diet.

Some diet books put so much emphasis on every single meal, causing their readers to become obsessed. A single meal they recommend requires a lot of preparation, and a trip to the grocery store. No one can stay on such an exhausting and time-consuming diet. Keep it simple! As long as you are sticking with the program most of the time (eighty percent), then the meals that you put extra effort into or go overboard on (twenty percent) will be much more appreciated and enjoyed.

JASON'S FORMULA

As a single professional, Jason works in an office five days a week where he takes thirty-minute lunch breaks in the company lunchroom. He's usually tired after a long day, heads home, and heats a dinner he prepared the previous weekend.

Maintaining a healthy weight has been a challenge since he was a child, considering his family was overweight. He grew up in a small town, and there wasn't much happening. So spontaneity with food, frequent restaurant eating, and encouragement to stuff oneself was the norm. It was their way of life.

When Jason got his degree and moved to the city, he was motivated to change. He realized he needed to give himself structure with his eating plan to keep himself on track. Here's what he does today to stay lean.

Most days, one meal is ground turkey and veggies. Every week, he simmers several pounds with sodium-free and fructose-free spaghetti sauce. He experiments with different spices each week. Examples are cumin with cayenne pepper, Italian herbs, and garlic with a bay leaf. The single servings are portioned into individual storage containers. Adding fresh carrots or cherry tomatoes in his cooler, he always has a quick, healthy meal ready to heat up at the office.

When he is at home, he has more time and leverage. He eats something similar, but instead of carrots, he adds frozen vegetables. He grabs a bag from the freezer, dumps some on a dinner plate, nukes them for three or so minutes, and then adds the lean meat for another minute.

While his meal heats, Jason doesn't rummage through the pantry for snacks to munch on before his dinner is ready. Instead, he goes through the mail or changes clothes. This small, yet intentional act helps Jason stay with his goals and his formula to eat better and lose weight.

Since he eats these same meals most days, he knows approximately how much turkey and how many veggies he will need. At his grocery store trip, he buys enough of these foods to last him for the entire week.

HOW OFTEN TO GROCERY SHOP?

It's better to take trips every two to three days rather than stock up on foods you'll overeat. It is also preferable to shop this way if you eat many dairy products, fresh meats you don't freeze, or seasonal produce.

Your lifestyle will also determine your shopping frequency, how many people you buy food for, and how convenient it is to get to the store.

I plan on one time a week, but I usually go two to three times because of things I forget. We live in an area where stores are close by, so I try to combine errands to save time. For example, I'll get gas, then swing by the shipping store, and drop by the grocery store—all in the same parking lot.

One great way to avoid temptation is to do your shopping online and either pick up your order or have it delivered to your home.

TRADITIONAL, ALL-IN-ONE, OR WAREHOUSE QUANTITY DISCOUNT STORE?

Let's look at all three of these. There are benefits and disadvantages to each.

Traditional grocery store: Usually smaller than the other two, these can make shopping quicker. If you like to save money, shop at several competing stores and compare prices. You might be surprised at what you find.

Another advantage of sticking with the same place is you know the layout of the store. You will be less likely to overlook or forget things on your normal list. You also probably won't have to backtrack through the store to find something, or track down an employee. What a headache that can be!

All-in-one supermarket: These stores have everything from yard tools, toys, clothing, food, and pet fish. They are usually big, but you can save big money if you shop only for those things you came for. Be sure to make your list and stick to it.

You might find their prices to be competitive with the traditional grocery stores—or even better.

Warehouse quantity discount store: Watch out before you decide this one is for you. Saving money is great. I love it! But will it be at the expense of you eating more? Try this option if you will, but keep a watch on your eating habits when you bring home huge bags, boxes, or containers of food you normally purchase in smaller amounts. This may be a temptation to eat more than you should.

YOUR PERSONAL GROCERY LIST ON YOUR MEAL PLAN

Don't underestimate the importance of a well-planned grocery list. Be aware that you can make poor choices there as easily as you can in a restaurant. You will most likely have a larger quantity of food to contend with at home, which could be a source of recurring temptation.

A good grocery list will give you the control you need. You make the decision to make good choices every day, but don't sabotage yourself at the grocery store. Don't go there hungry. Make a point to eat before you head out.

Most of you will want to plan for six meals each day—three meals and three snacks.

Your list will be based on your likes, dislikes, allergies, medical limitations, lifestyle, work schedule, and—above all—willingness.

Again, the following examples are not recommendations for your meals. Rather, they should only serve as a guide to designing your own formula, meal plan, and grocery list.

Before you prepare your list, decide on one or two foods you want to add, eliminate, or reduce. This decision will be part of your formula. Some examples could be to purchase more fiber-rich foods, eat fresh vegetables at least once a day, or switch from whole to two-percent or skim milk. List these ideas in your journal's section under "Goals."

Next, decide on one or two of your present behaviors to eliminate or change. Examples might be to read nutrition labels, stop eating at night, or quit buying crackers.

A great change for me was to focus on the fat content listed on the package. I made it my goal to avoid buying anything greater than twenty percent fat. Whatever you decide, list these in your journal.

It may take some time to determine what's important to you, so allow yourself space to develop this important step. Narrowing down your dietary priorities is the scaffolding from which your formula will be built. You will then be able to design the nutritional structure you desperately need.

Once you write down your goals, you will be able to make right selections. You've established your own personal boundaries. This is so much better than having someone else do it for you. Nobody except you has this plan. It's as individual as you are. *(Now, don't you feel special?)*

Please go slowly with all this. As I mentioned before, it's not good to make too many nutritional changes too quickly. To make things more manageable, limit your "absolutes" to one or two at the beginning. Once you establish the new habits you have chosen, you can personalize your formula further. As time goes on, you will find your nutrition becoming better and healthier.

A TIMESAVING HINT

Prepare a standard grocery list of those things you buy at the grocer's almost every time you go, and keep it in your wallet, phone, or paper coupon folder. Make changes as needed to accommodate your lifestyle. Every time you shop, you'll already know what to buy.

I keep my grocery list in the notes section of my phone and add or delete as I need things. My phone is always with me, so it's super-easy to update my list. I take it to the store, delete items when I place things in my cart, and feel a wonderful sense of accomplishment. If the store is out of an item or I overlook something, it will remain on my list for the next trip.

DETERMINE YOUR INDIVIDUAL MEALS

MEAL 1: Breakfast. This is your most important meal. It gets your metabolism going at the beginning of the day. Decide what's best for you in your lifestyle, but be sure to eat breakfast. I can't tell you how much whining I've heard over the years from clients who want to skip breakfast. Just tell yourself this is not an option. Keep an open mind, and you'll move forward.

If you have enough time most mornings, you might prepare cooked whole-grain cereal or eggs and toast.

Are you rushed, getting kids out the door, with no time for yourself? Decide now what you will eat. Will it be something quick, like yogurt and fruit, a bowl of cereal, or a bagel and protein drink? Plan to have a lot of quick and healthy "grab and go" foods on hand, and add all these items to your grocery list.

You may choose to have a breakfast bar and a banana on those mornings. An alternative breakfast could be one or two hardboiled eggs, a glass of milk in a travel mug, and a piece of fruit. On the weekends, you may wish to make a vegetable-turkey omelet or wheat pancakes.

After making these decisions, your grocery list will look something like this:

Breakfast, granola, and/or protein bars. One or two boxes. Extra bars will be for snacks, variety, or last-minute meals you forgot to plan. These are not too perishable and can easily be stored in the pantry or your drawer at work. It's better to buy too many of these, rather than too few. Since these will be combined with other things, try to get those that have:

- Roughly 200 calories
- Fewer than ten grams of sugar
- About as many protein grams as carbohydrate grams.

If you find one that has all these things, but is high in sugar grams, add a glass of skim milk. The milk protein will offset the sugar.

Bananas. A bunch of several. You may need to shop a couple of times a week unless you like spotty bananas.

Bagels, whole grain or wheat. They usually come in packages of six; however, if you are a connoisseur, you can also purchase a baker's dozen at a specialty shop and use a freezer bag to store the extras. If you decide to eliminate gluten, most grocery stores carry options.

Milk. One half to one gallon. Your goals will determine whether you purchase whole, two-percent, skim, soy, or some other kind. Skim has the highest protein per cup.

Eggs. One dozen.

Bread. Again, your goals will determine what kind of bread you purchase. There are many healthy types—sprouted grain, whole grain, whole wheat. White bread is not a good option! Or not purchasing bread at all might be your choice.

Non-stick spray or some kind of healthy oil for cooking.

Plastic to-go containers in a variety of sizes.

Travel mug, insulated, with a lid.

Wow, that was a long list! The good news is you won't have to buy all this every week.

MEAL 2: Snack. A snack is just that—a small meal, like a piece of fruit, a single serving of yogurt, an ounce of hard cheese, or a protein bar. The purpose of this meal is to hold your appetite in check until lunch (so you don't make bad choices and overeat) and to keep your metabolism going so your energy levels don't crater.

Examples of snacks are:

- Granola bars
- Small protein bars
- Rice cakes with low-sugar peanut butter or nut butter
- Part-skim mozzarella string cheese
- Glass of skim milk
- Large skim milk latte at the coffee shop (when ordered this way, it's like a mini-meal with a jolt)
- Handful of nuts or pumpkin seeds (These are calorie-dense, so keep the serving size small. I measure mine in one-

quarter cupfuls and put them in sealable plastic bags so I can grab one and go. I even keep several bags in my car in case I find myself hungry and away from home. These have proven to be lifesavers on countless occasions!)

- Generous bag of cherry tomatoes or other bite-sized veggies
- One or two hard-boiled egg with crackers
- Fruit, such as seedless grapes, citrus fruits, or berries

NO VENDING MACHINES, PLEASE!

Do you snack from vending machines? They are conveniently placed for people who plan poorly. By the time you make the decision to visit one for a snack, you will be vulnerable to temptation and will almost always make a poor selection. Don't go there at all, even if there is something "healthy" available. The other items may look too good for you to resist. Stay away from the *habit of purchasing* from them, so you won't risk making an unhealthy choice when you're hungry.

Plan ahead for your snack—perhaps a few nuts one day and a granola bar with a glass of milk on alternate days. Add these snacks to your list.

MEAL 3: Lunch. Here you are at lunchtime! Where do you eat—the office, at your house, or on the road? You're safest if you stay at home, because you have that fully stocked refrigerator and pantry from your regularly planned grocery store trips.

What about bringing your lunch to the office or eating it on the road?

Keep meals prepared in single-serving containers to prevent making bad decisions when you're hungry. If these are ready to eat, you can be on your way to eating healthy—no decisions necessary. You've probably learned by now that to make a last-minute choice when famished is dangerous.

Many offices have a kitchenette and/or microwave oven. These make it easy to have a healthy, satisfying meal. If you work in an office, you might bring a lunch container with chicken breast, rice, and broccoli to enjoy as a fantastic, nutritious, and satisfyingly hot, home-cooked meal.

Here are some good choices:

- **Bag of frozen chicken breasts, salmon, soy "mock" chicken, or whatever type of lean meat you like**
- **Broccoli, frozen or fresh** (or whatever veggie you like)
- **Rice, with or without seasoning**. The flavorings add zest with few calories, but a lot of sodium. If you use the seasoned rice, try cooking your meat and veggies with no salt. When the food is all in the container together, the rice will flavor everything else.

Now you have an example of a lunch that could be brought to the office.

You have the most control when you prepare your own food.

Again, you have the most control when you prepare your own food. Going to lunch with a group of co-workers could be more of a challenge, but it doesn't have to be. Before you leave, go online to glance at the menu. Decide at that point what you will order. Simply choose the best item on the menu based on your formula. Stick with your plan. This will keep you on track with your goals.

At some lunch events, you won't be able to choose the caterer or restaurant. If you attend too many of these, you may find temptation a difficult struggle. My suggestion is to do the best you can. Your honesty, willingness, and support from friends will take you a long way.

Be prepared for the unexpected. For the rest of your life, you will encounter surprises. My goal in writing this book is to equip and empower you to anticipate and plan for these curve balls.

Sometimes you will be fully prepared. At other times, you won't even know what hit you. You'll just make the best of those situations, learn from your mistakes, and move on.

Finally, you're done with lunch. That was a long one!

MEAL 4: Snack. Now, suppose you're at the office. Do you get that sleepy, dragged-out feeling around 2:30 or 3:00? You might need a pick-me-up. Why not enjoy a snack, like a **low-fat blueberry muffin and cup of coffee**? Or, if carbohydrates make you drowsy, choose a higher protein snack, like a **part-skim mozzarella cheese stick and some whole grain crackers, nuts, or a cup of yogurt**. This is a snack, remember, so keep it small. Let's say you opt for the muffin.

Here's the grocery list now:

- **Low fat blueberry muffins**. One or two four-pack containers from the bakery (some will go into the freezer to keep fresh). You might try your hand at homemade muffins or store-bought mixes, which are so much cheaper. Making them at home gives you more control over what goes in them. Just look at the recipe and add those ingredients to your grocery list.

- **Cheese sticks**. Part-skim mozzarella

- **Whole grain crackers**

- **Yogurt, plain and non-fat**. Single-sized containers. You can add sweetener, cinnamon, and/or vanilla extract. Be creative! Cocoa, carob, and other extracts are also delicious with plain yogurt.

At 4:00 or 5:00 p.m., your office day is over (hopefully). Did you pack your workout bag with your shoes and workout clothes? The easiest way to get your gym time in is while traveling from one place to another.

What better time to go than after work, where the exercise helps you decompress from the day's stress. You should be well-fueled from regular meals throughout the day, so your energy will be high. Have a great workout! And if you need a small snack first, carry one with you to eat as you travel to the gym. Don't forget to add it to your grocery list.

MEAL 5: Dinner. By the time you get home from the gym, you'll definitely be hungry, but not famished. You'll be in control and completely capable of making sound nutritional decisions. If you have prepared well, there will be something quick and easy waiting for you in the refrigerator to heat and eat.

If you're comfortable with Jason's plan (above), you can eat something similar. Other examples of dinners could be chicken breast, fish, or soy meat with a salad and vegetables. You could even throw together a Crockpot meal of meat and vegetables in the morning before leaving the house. What a wonderful aroma to welcome you home!

MEAL 6: Snack. Later in the evening, you may be surprised to find that you're hungry. Eat something you have on hand (yogurt, piece of fruit, or low-carbohydrate protein drink). Find what works for you at that time of day to help you wind down and relax. Perhaps it's simply a cup of hot, decaffeinated herbal tea. Maybe nothing at all.

Be careful about your carbohydrate intake at night. If you want to lose body fat, it's better to choose a higher-protein snack, rather than a starchy one. A glass of **whey protein** mixed with water or milk, a hard-boiled egg, or an ounce of cheese would all be good choices.

Here's the final list. Are you happy with yours? If not, make changes now, before going to the store. When you're there, you'll most likely make more changes, based on the information you learn on those nutrition labels. Don't forget your calculator!

- Breakfast, granola, and/or protein bars, one or two boxes
- Bananas
- Bagels
- Milk
- Fruit
- Eggs
- Whole grain bread
- Non-stick spray and/or oil
- Plastic to-go containers, silverware, napkins
- Car coffee cup with lid
- Nuts
- A variety of lean, fresh meats
- Vegetables
- Rice
- Coffee, cream, and/or sugar-free sweetener
- Low-fat muffins, package of four
- Jar of spaghetti sauce
- Spices, salt and pepper
- Yogurt, single-sized containers
- Whey protein powder. (Health food stores have a variety of these. You may even find one you like in your grocery store. Save more money by buying in quantity or on sale.)

A NOTE ON SUPPLEMENTS

Did you know that the supplement industry is not regulated like the food and drug industry?[xiii] Because of this, the labeling is not consistent. You'll find some information on one brand, but you may not be able to compare it to other brands. If you do use protein drinks or other meal supplements, try to choose a brand from a reputable company, one that has been around for a few years. If you're still unsure as to which one is best, ask someone with experience what he or she chooses.

This information should help you formulate your own meal plan, based on your unique life and individuality. I'm sure you will have challenges I've not mentioned here, and I would love to hear about your experiences as you venture forward on your own journey toward better health. Don't hesitate to employ a nutritionist or dietician if you need more help with portion sizes or other specifics. It will be money well spent, even if it's only one session.

Don't rely on novices to tell you what to eat. Following another's plan will only reap temporary results, if at all. Your diet prescription and ultimate formula need to come from you (and your professional, if you use one). At first, this will require more work, but it will become an integral part of you.

Your formula is your own, to grow and change for the rest of your life. It can and will work for you.

CONCLUSION

Your formula will not only consist of specific food items to add to or omit from your diet, but it will also include adding or eliminating certain behaviors. In fact, if you change your eating habits, this may be as important to your success as what you eat.

It is so easy to eat too much from original containers. You may have to eat differently if you tend to enjoy eating directly from bags, tubs, or boxes of food.

To help you control portioning, when you get home from the grocery store, immediately take care of this problem. Open whatever food you want to separate. Get some snack-sized plastic bags, and immediately and evenly redistribute the whole package. Toss the original container.

If you struggle with portion control, don't fail to divvy up those foods when you are feeling strong. The day you forget may be the day you eat the whole package.

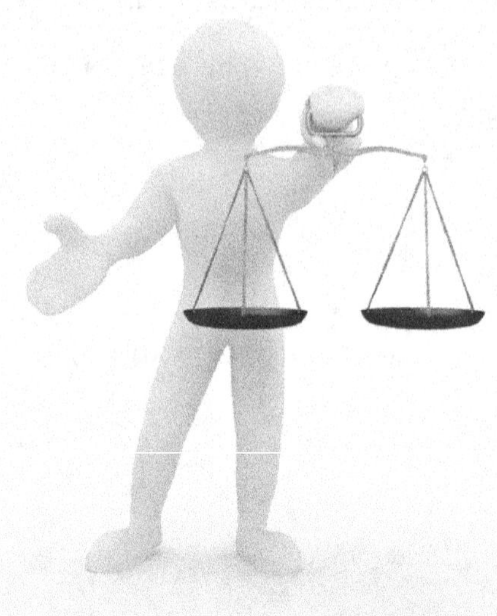

18. NUTRITION LABEL COMPARISON

"Information is a source of learning. But unless it is organized, processed, and available to the right people in a format for decision making it is a burden, not a benefit." —William Pollard

You just got finished with your grocery list, so now let's look at nutrition labels. What do these labels tell you? How can you read them so you benefit the most from your goals?

Don't look only at the images and words of a product to get information about what's inside. You are deceiving yourself if you do, because these pictures and text may or may not be an accurate description of what's in the item.

"What?" you say. "Do you mean to tell me the food company could be lying to me on the front of the box?"

Yes, I am. In fact, I am saying the manufacturer could be trying to deceive and/or manipulate you. They may be trying to keep the truth from you regarding their product. They want it to taste good so you'll buy it again. But they may not want you to know how they got it to taste so good.

The goal of any food company is to sell. The labeling on the front of a container is for marketing purposes only. These labels are masterfully designed to attract attention in order to move as much of that product as possible.

The facts are found on the nutrition label on the back of the container. At least, that's usually where you'll find them. (On rare occasions, there is no nutrition label.) Once you understand how to decipher this information, you will be capable of making better decisions.

I also want to mention that in some of the examples in this chapter, the data on the manufacturer's label was not entirely accurate. For example, fat has nine calories per gram, but there were cases where I noticed the fat calories per serving were not equal to the fat grams multiplied by nine. My job here is not to police these manufacturers but to help you maximize your results. So I warn you to always do the calculations for the best results.

You must know what you're eating.

You must know what you're eating. You need to know the cause of why you are or are not getting the results you seek. One reason why you've failed to reach your goals in the past may be because you never had accurate information in the first place. You might have thought you knew what you were eating, but chances are you didn't.

Taking the grocery list above, you'll see each item in this section. There will be two examples of comparable items. This comparison will help you consider both products and make a decision for yourself. The actual brands and package designs have been omitted to allow you to focus only on the nutritional content.

I'll make one or two observations from each example to draw your attention to the products' differences. By the time you're finished, you should be able to base your food purchases on what you learn from the nutrition labels.

It's best to buy foods that are as close to their natural state as possible. That is how God made our food for us. Doing so will help you keep your diet healthy. You can't go wrong by keeping it simple. However, lower your expectations about perfectly adhering to your ideals. You'll find this to be somewhat of a juggling game. What do I mean by this? Well, if something is a bit higher in sugar than you like, combine it with something low in sugar and protein-packed. If you eat something higher in fat than you normally consume, eat less fat than usual the rest of the day.

GRANOLA BARS[xiv] VS. TOASTER PASTRIES[xv]

Granola Bar, Oats and Honey		Toaster Pastry, Frosted Brown Sugar Cinnamon	
Serving Size: 2 bars (42g)		Serving Size: 1 pastry (50g)	
Amount Per Serving		Amount Per Serving	
Calories 190 Calories From Fat 60		**Calories** 210 Calories From Fat 60	
Total Fat	6 g	**Total Fat**	7g
Saturated Fat .5 g Trans Fat 0 g		Saturated Fat 2.5 g Trans Fat 0 g	
Cholesterol	0 mg	**Cholesterol**	0 mg
Sodium	160 mg	**Sodium**	170 mg
Total Carbohydrates	29 g	**Total Carbohydrates**	35 g
Dietary Fiber 2 g Sugars 12 g		Dietary Fiber <1 g Sugars 15 g	
Protein	4 g	**Protein**	2 g

Granola bars and toaster pastries typically come in wrapped

packages of two, but the serving size on the label differs for this example. If you notice the grams, they are fairly close for two granola bars and one pastry, so this is how we'll compare them. By the way, if you eat toaster pastries, do you only eat one? If not, you'll need to double these numbers to see what you're consuming.

Do you remember the list of two items you want to eliminate or improve on your diet? Well, lowering fat calories should be on the list of anyone who wants to lose weight. In fact, deciding to limit your total fat calories to twenty-five to thirty-five percent of your total intake is probably an ideal rule to follow. If you purchase most products that fall within this range, your chances of losing weight are greater.

Limit your total fat calories to 25-35% of your total intake.

Follow this maximum fat percentage rule here as you look at labels to be considered within a "low fat" range. Let's now see how much fat is in each of these items.

It might be difficult to know how much fat is in a food item simply by glancing at the label. In order to know exactly how much fat you are eating as a percentage, use the following calculation:

$$\frac{\text{Calories From Fat Per Serving}}{\text{Total Calories Per Serving}} = \% \text{ Fat}$$

For the granola bars, this calculation will be 60/190 = 32% fat. The pastries will be 60/210 = 29% fat. The granola bars are slightly more in fat than the pastry.

These two labels have some minor variations, but the real differences will be found in the ingredient listings. Check these out:

Granola Bar Ingredients: *Whole grain oats, sugar, canola oil, yellow corn flour, honey, soy flour, brown sugar syrup, salt, soy lecithin, baking soda, natural flavor.*

Toaster Pastry Ingredients: *Enriched flour (wheat flour, niacin, reduced iron, vitamin B1 [thiamine mononitrate], vitamin B2 [riboflavin], folic acid), sugar, soybean and palm oil (with TBHQ for freshness), corn syrup, dextrose, high fructose corn syrup, cracker meal, contains two percent or less of molasses, salt, calcium carbonate, leavening (baking soda, sodium acid pyrophosphate, monocalcium phosphate), cinnamon, wheat starch, gelatin, caramel color, soy lecithin, vitamin A palmitate, niacinamide, reduced iron, vitamin B6 (pyridoxine hydrochloride), vitamin B2 (riboflavin), vitamin B1 (thiamin hydrochloride).*

If you had stopped with the nutrition label, you may have chosen either one. Now that you've seen the ingredients, what would your choice be?

Is this information surprising to you? Now that you know this, which would you choose? Remember, neither is an option.

CONCLUSION

These products' labels were roughly the same, but maybe not nutritionally so. Does it matter to you if a product has naturally occurring nutrients or if the nutrients have been added by the manufacturer? If you need more information to make your decision, look at the rest of the label and also the ingredients. You can also contact the manufacturer.

I encourage you to look for alternatives to explore for your grocery list. Carry a pen, paper, and calculator with you to the grocery store. If you don't know what some ingredient means, you can always write it down and look it up later.

BAGELS: RESTAURANT[xvi] AND GROCERY STORE[xvii]

Bagel #1, Restaurant		Bagel #2, Grocery Store	
Serving Size: 1 Bagel		Serving Size: 1 bagel (95g)	
Amount Per Serving		Amount Per Serving	
Calories 330 Calories From Fat		**Calories** 260 Calories From Fat 10	
Total Fat	2 g	**Total Fat**	1 g
Saturated Fat 0 g Trans Fat 0 g		Saturated Fat 0 g Trans Fat 0 g	
Cholesterol	0 mg	**Cholesterol**	0 mg
Sodium	760 mg	**Sodium**	400 mg
Total Carbohydrates	70 g	**Total Carbohydrates**	50 g
Dietary Fiber 3 g Sugars 6 g		Dietary Fiber 2 g Sugars 3 g	
Protein	12 g	**Protein**	9 g

For the restaurant bagel, I obtained the data from an outside source and not a label. The first thing I noticed about these bagels was the apparent size difference. Although the grams are not given for the restaurant bagel, you can look at the other information and know it's bigger: calories, sodium, and carbohydrates are all significantly more.

I'll show you more detail on carbohydrates in Formula Buster #15, but for now, consider carbs as energy. And since there's little fiber to offset these carb grams, the energy enters your bloodstream quickly, a process which doesn't bode well for those trying to lose weight.

CONCLUSION

In this example, you would do less damage by selecting the smaller bagel. Doing so may not be realistic when you're sitting in the restaurant, but as long as you know what you're consuming, you'll understand why you are or are not you are getting the results you want.

One Sunday morning when I was single, I bought a baker's dozen

(13) of bagels. Throughout that day, I ate nothing but bagels—nine of them! I like to tell this story to tell people about how sneaky my cravings were. I didn't even realize what I had done until they were almost gone.

I don't know if I craved those bagels because they were hot and chewy or simply because they were a processed bread product. What I do know is I can't eat a bagel today unless I combine it with a glass of whey protein, an egg, or a glass of skim milk. The protein from those items offsets the carbohydrate, so I'm less likely to crave another one. The most important thing for me is to only purchase one bagel at a time, instead of several or more. It's more expensive this way, but I'll only eat one.

COCONUT MILK[xviii] *VS.* 2% MILK[xix]

Coconut Milk		2% Milk	
Serving Size: 1/4 cup (60 ml)		Serving Size: 1 cup (240 ml)	
Amount Per Serving		Amount Per Serving	
Calories 142 Calories From Fat 118		**Calories** 130 Calories From Fat 63	
Total Fat	13.1 g	**Total Fat**	8 g
Saturated Fat 11.6 g Trans Fat 0 g		Saturated Fat 16 g Trans Fat 0 g	
Cholesterol	0 mg	**Cholesterol**	20 mg
Sodium	37 mg	**Sodium**	120 mg
Total Carbohydrates	6 g	**Total Carbohydrates**	12 g
Dietary Fiber 1.6 g Sugars 4.6 g		Dietary Fiber 0 g Sugars 12 g	
Protein	4 g	**Protein**	9 g

Here is an example of a serving size discrepancy. Notice that the calories are similar (142 and 130) for each product per serving.

However, look closer. One serving is *two ounces* (quarter cup) for the coconut milk and *eight ounces* (one whole cup) for the milk. Do you wonder why the manufacturer of the coconut milk did this? I suspect they attempted to make the labels as comparable as possible in order to sell more coconut milk. A potential buyer might look at the calories and think, "Oh, this is about the same as the milk I drink. I'll buy this instead."

Looking closer, the coconut milk has almost *four times* the calories as the milk. I get this number by multiplying 142 by four, since there are four two-ounce servings in each cup of milk.

Now, who is going to have a two-ounce glass of coconut milk? Maybe if you wanted to taste it. Most people would have a normal-sized glass, unknowingly consuming 568 calories and 83% fat! Here's the fat calculation for the coconut milk:

$$\frac{\textbf{118 Fat Calories Per Serving}}{\textbf{142 Calories Per Serving}} = \textbf{83\% Calories From Fat}$$

And there's one more thing about the coconut milk: it has an emulsifier in it (guar gum). An emulsifier is necessary because there is so much fat in the coconut milk; the product would separate if the emulsifier weren't in it.

The two-percent milk is not a low-fat product either, but it seems low by comparison:

$$\frac{\textbf{63 Fat Calories Per Serving}}{\textbf{130 Calories Per Serving}} = \textbf{48\% Calories From Fat}$$

CONCLUSION

This example serves as a warning to always pay attention to everything on the nutrition label on the back of the product. Would you buy this if you knew you were drinking almost 500 calories of a 75% fat product? You may, depending on your absolutes you determined earlier. For example, if you want to eat a cholesterol-free or vegetarian diet, the coconut milk may be a better choice.

WHITE[xx] *VS.* SPROUTED GRAIN BREAD[xxi]

White Bread		Sprouted Grain Bread	
Serving Size: 1 slice (28g)		Serving Size: 1 slice (34g)	
Amount Per Serving		Amount Per Serving	
Calories 70 Calories From Fat 5		**Calories** 80 Calories From Fat 10	
Total Fat	0.5 g	**Total Fat**	1 g
Saturated Fat 0 g Trans Fat 0 g		Saturated Fat 0 g Trans Fat 0 g	
Cholesterol	0 mg	**Cholesterol**	0 mg
Sodium	160 mg	**Sodium**	70 mg
Total Carbohydrates	15 g	**Total Carbohydrates**	14 g
Dietary Fiber < 1 g Sugars 3 g		Dietary Fiber 4 g Sugars 0 g	
Protein	2 g	**Protein**	5 g

White Bread Ingredients*: Enriched unbleached flour (wheat flour, malted barley flour, niacin, reduced iron, thiamine mononitrate, riboflavin, folic acid), water, sugar, yeast, contains less than 2% of the following: soybean oil, salt, calcium propionate (preservative), dough conditioners (sodium stearoyl lactylate, monoglycerides, enzymes, ascorbic acid), monocalcium phosphate, calcium sulfate.*

Sprouted Grain Bread Ingredients*: Organic sprouted wheat, filtered water, organic sprouted flax, organic sprouted barley, organic sprouted millet, organic malted barley, organic sprouted lentils, organic sprouted soybeans, organic sprouted spelt, fresh yeast, organic wheat gluten, sea salt, rolled in organic flax seeds.*

When you see things like calcium propionate[xxii] and stearoyl lactylate[xxiii] do you wonder, "What in the world are these?"; or "Can they be bad for my body?"; and "What's the long-term impact of this stuff to my health?"; or "What would the product look like—and how would it taste—if it only had natural components?"

The sprouted grain includes simple ingredients. I can imagine my mother making this type of bread when I was a child.

"But the white bread tastes so good," you declare. I totally understand. It's so hard to think about giving up something to which you have a strong attachment. In fact, certain food items conjure up positive emotional memories. It seems a betrayal to ourselves to let go of certain things. They have become a tradition in our daily lives. Statements like, "I have a right to eat ________" or "I am entitled to have __________" come to mind.

Will you try something? You most likely have enough information to make the best choice between these two items. Use your knowledge to control your desire. In fact, don't try to adjust your craving, and don't even think about it. Simply use your head. Because when you combat an emotional urge with thought, you're bound to lose. Let's just ignore it, and work with your mind in another way.

If you know in your heart that something isn't good for you, try to at least transition away from it. Move toward a healthier alternative. For example, if you're a white-bread lover, you can buy half-white or half-wheat for a few weeks, then try wheat. Experiment with different brands. The store bakery will also have nutritious, freshly baked breads.

This example shows two extremes. Perhaps you stopped eating white bread years ago and only eat whole wheat these days. If that's the case, start noticing the ingredients on the labels of the foods you currently eat. They may have changed since the last time you looked. You might be surprised at what you find. You also might decide to stop eating something you have been enjoying for years because you know more about that product today.

CONCLUSION

Here again is an example of similar nutrition labels with huge differences in the ingredients. At first glance, these items seem to have roughly the same values. However, there is a larger difference in nutritional value.

When you choose one item over another, don't be fooled to think these products are the same, simply because many numbers are similar. Always opt for the higher nutrition, except when a medical issue dictates that you stay away from certain foods.

Your body was created to work, and this includes your digestive tract. Choose foods with higher fiber and you'll stay healthier and leaner.

The quickest way to reach your goals is by making consistently better choices over a period of time. Like a beautiful sculpture created by multiple chisels, good nutrition is a process of chipping away at the old habits and forming new ones. It's a way of life, and it will always be changing.

PUMPKIN SEEDS[xxiv] VS. CINNAMON PECANS[xxv]

White Pumpkin Seeds, Roasted and Salted		Cinnamon Pecans	
Serving Size: 1 oz (28g)		Serving Size: 20 pieces (28 g)	
Amount Per Serving		Amount Per Serving	
Calories 148 Calories From Fat 108		**Calories** 190 Calories From Fat 150	
Total Fat	12 g	**Total Fat**	17 g
Saturated Fat 2 g Trans Fat 0 g		Saturated Fat 1.5 g Trans Fat 0 g	
Cholesterol	0 mg	**Cholesterol**	0 mg
Sodium	163 mg	**Sodium**	55 mg
Total Carbohydrates	4 g	**Total Carbohydrates**	8 g
Dietary Fiber 1 g Sugars 1 g		Dietary Fiber 2 g Sugars 5 g	
Protein	9 g	**Protein**	2 g

Seeds or nuts? Which do you prefer? They are all healthy and nutrient-dense. What could cause us to choose one over the other?

The first thing to notice is the serving size: one-quarter cup or approximately one ounce. Do you know how small this is? Have you ever purchased a package or bag of anything and consumed its contents without considering the serving size? I sure have. I was in for some rude awakenings when I started making those calculations. You may find the same is true for you.

Many of you might be surprised to find that one ounce of nuts or seeds is plenty for a meal. If you aren't sure about this, then for one time only, eat that amount of the nuts/seeds and see how you feel in about 20 to 30 minutes.

The pecans have two protein grams to offset a higher amount of sugar (5 g) and carbohydrates (8 g). When you have this type of situation and add high fat, it's a bad choice for anyone who wants to lose weight. Why? Because your blood sugar will spike and all that fat will be swept into your fat stores. Even though these amounts are small, there are too few protein grams to balance them. This scenario may cause you to crave more and overeat.

The seeds have nine protein grams with fewer sugar (1 g), fat (12 g), and carbohydrates (4 g). This combination will be more satisfying and won't cause unwanted cravings.

CONCLUSION

The last thing you want to do is eat something, and then soon after have it calling your name. Once that irresistible craving sets in, you're a goner. You must be vigilant about your choices if you want to succeed, because once you eat something that doesn't agree with you, you may suffer some consequences.

Almost all types of nuts and seeds are high in fat. This is why the portion sizes are so small. It doesn't take a lot to make a full meal. Also, although these are healthy things to eat, many people choose to avoid them because they lose control and eat too much. However, this shouldn't stop you from eating them and gaining those great nutritional benefits they offer.

SKINLESS CHICKEN BREAST[xxvi] *VS.* TERIYAKI CHICKEN BREAST[xxvii]

Skinless Chicken Breast		Teriyaki Chicken Breast	
Serving Size: ½ breast (~4 oz or 112 g)		Serving Size: 1 piece (139 g)	
Amount Per Serving		Amount Per Serving	
Calories 130 Calories From Fat 13		Calories 180 Calories From Fat 20	
Total Fat	1.5 g	**Total Fat**	2 g
Saturated Fat 0.4 g Trans Fat 0 g		Saturated Fat 0.5 g Trans Fat 0 g	
Cholesterol	68 mg	**Cholesterol**	70 mg
Sodium	77 mg	**Sodium**	560 mg
Total Carbohydrates	0 g	**Total Carbohydrates**	8 g
Dietary Fiber 0 g Sugars 0 g		Dietary Fiber 0 g Sugars 5 g	
Protein	27 g	**Protein**	31 g

Below is the fat calculation for the regular chicken breast:

13 / 130 = 10% calories from fat

And from the seasoned chicken breast:

20 / 180 = 11% calories from fat

CONCLUSION

Carbohydrates and total calories are slightly higher for the teriyaki chicken, possibly due to the seasoning. These two labels are comparable with the exception of sodium, obviously from the seasoning. There's a big difference between both examples here. If sodium isn't a problem for you, either one of these items should be acceptable.

LEAN GROUND TURKEY[xxviii] *VS.* EXTRA LEAN GROUND[xxix] TURKEY

Lean Ground Turkey		Extra Lean Ground Turkey	
Serving Size: 4 oz (112 g)		Serving Size: 4 oz (112 g)	
Amount Per Serving		Amount Per Serving	
Calories 170 Calories From Fat 70		**Calories** 120 Calories From Fat 15	
Total Fat	8 g	**Total Fat**	1.5 g
Saturated Fat 2.5 g Trans Fat 0 g		Saturated Fat 0.5 g Trans Fat 0 g	
Cholesterol	80 mg	**Cholesterol**	55 mg
Sodium	80 mg	**Sodium**	70 mg
Total Carbohydrates	0 g	**Total Carbohydrates**	0 g
Dietary Fiber 0 g Sugars 0 g		Dietary Fiber 0 g Sugars 0 g	
Protein	21 g	**Protein**	26 g

You may see "93% Lean 7% Fat" on the front label of a lean ground turkey label. "Lean,"[xxx] in the meat-packing industry, is defined as a product with less than 10% fat *by weight*. This is not to be confused with 10% fat *by calories*. But you might assume that since the product says "lean" on the front of the package, it is in fact, a lean product. But this would not necessarily be correct, as you'll see in this comparison.

This is an example of the deceptiveness on the part of the meat-packing industry to sell their product.

So how "lean" is this ground turkey? Let's find out.

70/170 = 41% calories from fat

Now look at the extra-lean label and do that calculation:

15/120 = 13% calories from fat

By the way, it doesn't matter what the serving size is when you do this fat calculation. The percentage will be constant regardless of the quantity consumed. If your aim is for most products to be 25-35% fat calories or less, this will be the only calculation you will have to do on products containing fat. In other words, a four-ounce serving of the lean ground turkey will have the same percentage of fat (41%) as an eight-ounce serving, and a four-ounce serving of the extra lean ground turkey will have the same percentage of fat (13%) as an eight-ounce serving.

CONCLUSION

Be aware of the ways you can be fooled by labels. Always be on the safe side by checking the nutrition label on the back of the product and working your calculations.

FRESH BROCCOLI[xxxi] *VS.* BROCCOLI WITH CHEESE[xxxii]

Fresh Broccoli		Broccoli with Cheese Sauce	
Serving Size: 3 ½ oz (100 g)		Serving Size: 2/3 c (110 g)	
Amount Per Serving		Amount Per Serving	
Calories 34 Calories From Fat 0		**Calories** 60 Calories From Fat 18	
Total Fat	0 g	**Total Fat**	2 g
Saturated Fat 0 g Trans Fat 0 g		Saturated Fat 1 g Trans Fat 0 g	
Cholesterol	0 mg	**Cholesterol**	5 mg
Sodium	33 mg	**Sodium**	430 mg
Total Carbohydrates	7 g	**Total Carbohydrates**	7 g
Dietary Fiber 3 g Sugars 2 g		Dietary Fiber 1 g Sugars 2 g	
Protein	3 g	**Protein**	2 g

Here is an example of what happens when a lot of "goop" is added to a basically healthy product. The cheese version has fat, more than twice as many calories, and more than *ten times* the amount sodium of fresh broccoli.

Many people believe fresh vegetables are always the best choice. But suppose they have to be transported quite a distance before arriving to the grocery store, then to your house, and finally to your stove. This is true for a lot of produce.

For example, in my neighborhood grocery stores, I recall seeing produce from California, Chile, and Mexico on a regular basis. I'm sure there are more origins than those. So if you are opting to maximize the nutrients in the fresh vegetables and fruits you buy, you may be better off purchasing those that are locally grown.

Surprisingly, frozen vegetables might be more healthful to eat than the fresh. Because when they come out of the field, they're washed, cut, packaged, and frozen. This quick process locks in the nutrients.

Canned vegetables are already cooked prior to canning, and are usually reheated before eating. All this cook time leaches out nutrients, so you won't receive as much nutritional benefit compared to fresh or frozen.

CONCLUSION

Fresh and frozen veggies are more nutritionally ideal than canned, but consider your lifestyle first. Are you going to spend the time required to wash, cut, and prepare fresh produce? Is it easier to buy the more expensive pre-packaged products and skip some of the work? Can you afford to do this consistently? Or, would you prefer to buy only frozen?

Although canned vegetables are not the best *nutritional* choice, if you won't eat them otherwise, they may be *your* best choice.

WHITE,[xxxiii] WILD,[xxxiv] AND BROWN RICE[xxxv] (COOKED)

White Rice, Enriched		Wild Rice		Brown Rice	
Serving:	1 cup	Serving:	1 cup	Serving:	1 cup
Calories	199	Calories	166	Calories	216
Fat	0.4 g	Fat	0.6 g	Fat	1.8 g
Sodium	7 mg	Sodium	5 mg	Sodium	10 mg
Carbs	45 g	Carbs	35 g	Carbs	45 g
Dietary Fiber	1.2 g	Dietary Fiber	3 g	Dietary Fiber	3.5 g
Protein	4.2 g	Protein	7 g	Protein	5 g

Any time you see the word "enriched" on bread, rice, and other cereal packaging, all the naturally occurring nutrients have been stripped from the product. In their place, the manufacturer added man-made components. So if you compare the labels on these three types of rice, you might think they are equally nutritious.

Brown rice is whole grain rice, un-milled, with the inedible outer hull removed. The bran, germ, and endosperm are left intact. White rice is the same grain with the hull, bran layer, and cereal germ removed.

CONCLUSION

All three rice varieties have minor differences of calories, fat, sodium, and carbohydrates. But there is more fiber and protein in the brown and wild rice.

Selecting brown over wild rice or vice versa will be a matter of preference or budget (wild rice tends to be the most expensive of the three). Often, you'll see a combination of brown and wild rice at the store.

Nothing compares to natural food. God made it this way, perfectly tailored for our physical needs. We are wise to keep our food choices as simple as possible.

HALF-AND-HALF[xxxvi] *VS.* POWDERED PLAIN NON-DAIRY CREAMER[xxxvii]

Half And Half		Powdered Non-Dairy Creamer	
Serving Size: 1 tablespoon (15 g)		Serving Size: 1 teaspoon (2g)	
Amount Per Serving		Amount Per Serving	
Calories 20 Calories From Fat 15		**Calories** 10 Calories From Fat 5	
Total Fat	1.7 g	**Total Fat**	0.5 g
Saturated Fat 1.1 g Trans Fat 0 g		Saturated Fat 0.5 g Trans Fat 0 g	
Cholesterol	6 mg	**Cholesterol**	0 mg
Sodium	6 mg	**Sodium**	0 mg
Total Carbohydrates	0.6 g	**Total Carbohydrates**	1 g
Dietary Fiber 0 g Sugars 0 g		Dietary Fiber Sugars	
Protein	0.4 g	**Protein**	0 g

I have tried countless times to eliminate, cut back, or modify the cream in my coffee, hoping to save some calories, lower my fat intake, or improve my nutrition. If you're like me, you'd rather not have coffee if you can't have it your way. So if you insist on having cream with your coffee, this comparison is for you.

If you are trying to lose weight, changing the way you drink coffee could help substantially, depending on how many cups you drink each day. Consider and try any possible creamer alternatives that are attractive to you. You will find milk-based, soy-based, and others completely artificial. Make your decision based on the information you find, along with your personal preferences.

Much of what you decide to eat or drink will be a tradeoff. For example, there may be chemicals in non-dairy creamer, but if you're a vegetarian, you may choose to use this anyway.

On the other hand, you may prefer half-and-half in your coffee and eat less fat throughout the day to compensate for the added calories.

Both of these creamer examples below are high in fat: 75% for the half-and-half, and 50% for the creamer. The question is, regardless of which you choose, how *much* do you put in one cup of coffee? Let's find out.

For half-and-half users, notice the serving size is one tablespoon. Next time you have a cup and before you add it to your coffee, pour the liquid into a tablespoon before adding it to the cup. Count the number you add and get a total, multiplied by the number of cups you drink. The powdered creamer will be done the same way. However, the serving size is one *teaspoon*. Make sure the product is level and not heaping so you have an accurate volume. Count the number of spoons you add.

Calculate the total calories you are consuming for each cup of coffee, based on what the label says and your servings consumed. For the half-and-half, if you have four tablespoons in each of two cups, you are consuming eight tablespoons. This would equal 160 calories and 120 fat calories. Once you realize how much you're consuming, you may change to another creamer. But this pales in comparison to what you'll see next.

Now let's consider sugar. Many coffee creamers are loaded with it. By looking at the nutrition labels in these examples, you can see that each product has little or no sugar listed. This is true for the half-and-half, which is a blend of equal parts whole milk and light cream. Any sugar present from lactose is very low.

But wait! Look now at the ingredients for the powdered non-dairy creamer:

Powdered Plain Non-Dairy Creamer Ingredients: *Corn syrup solids, hydrogenated vegetable oil (coconut and/or palm kernel and/or soybean), sodium caseinate (a milk derivative)**, less than 2% Of dipotassium phosphate, mono- and diglycerides, sodium aluminosilicate, artificial flavor, annatto color. **Not A Source Of Lactose*

In any product, ingredients are listed in order, from the greatest to the least. And we see the first is corn syrup solids, which is another name for sugar. Something isn't right here. If this is the number one ingredient, how can the sugar not even be listed on the nutrition label? How does the manufacturer get away with that?

Another indication of a discrepancy is that five out of ten calories per serving are fat calories, but where do the other five come from? Also note, there is one gram of carbohydrate indicated (there are four calories in each gram from carbs).

The other five calories are coming from somewhere, so if half of them come from the fat, the other half must be sugar, since corn syrup solids is the primary ingredient. This label-flaw must be from a loophole, but don't be fooled. This product is one-half fat and one-half sugar.

So how do you know how much fat and sugar you are drinking with the non-dairy creamer? When you measured the amount you put in your coffee, you had a good idea of how much you put in each cup.

Suppose you drink two cups of coffee each morning and you use ten teaspoons of creamer in each cup of coffee or twenty teaspoons of creamer. That would mean you are consuming 200 calories (20 x 10 calories per teaspoon) with 100 calories fat and 100 calories sugar (approximately 25 grams of sugar). Now, *that's* an eye-opener!

CONCLUSION

Are you surprised to see something so innocuous as coffee creamer turn into a monster? As you persist with informing yourself about the foods you eat and drink, you will continue to have these types of revelations. This is good and exactly the thing that will help you reach the results you seek.

A NOTE ON CHOLESTEROL[xxxviii xxxix xl]

Cholesterol is a waxy, fat-like substance found in all cells of the body. It travels through the bloodstream in small packages called lipoproteins, and it can harden arteries and increase the risk of a heart attack. The Centers for Disease Control and Prevention estimate that almost thirty-two percent of American adults have high cholesterol.[xli]

While our bodies manufacture these substances, they are also found in animal products we eat—meat, butter, and cheese, for example. You need to watch the amount of fat you consume, especially saturated fat, which comes mostly from animal products. The cholesterol in your body comes from your diet and what your body manufactures.

Exercise helps to lower your cholesterol because it burns fat. The habit of regular physical activity is like taking out insurance against all kinds of ailments—heart disease caused by high cholesterol being only one of them.

If you are unsure as to how much fat to eat, how much saturated fat to avoid, or you have confusion about all of this, you are not alone. What I've stressed here is the principle of keeping your fat intake no greater than twenty-five to thirty-five percent of total daily calories. If you want more information on fat intake, do some online investigating or schedule a session with a nutritionist.

What you monitor in your diet will be up to you, based on your physical needs, medical issues (if any), medications you might be on, or anything else that may determine whether or not you eat or limit certain things.

It is possible to control your cholesterol exclusively with a healthy diet and exercise program, using no medication. I've seen clients get off their cholesterol medication completely by changing their diet and adding regular workouts.

One client lowered hers by taking a red yeast rice supplement she got at the health food store. This contains a natural statin, which has been proven to lower cholesterol.

CHOCOLATE CHIP MUFFIN:
CONVENIENCE STORE[xlii] *VS.* MIX[xliii]

Convenience Store Muffin	Muffin Mix, Prepared with Water
Serving Size: 1/3 muffin (52 g)	Serving Size: 1 muffin (31 g)
Amount Per Serving	Amount Per Serving
Calories 200 Calories From Fat 100	**Calories** 120 Calories From Fat 30
Total Fat 11 g	**Total Fat** 3 g
Saturated Fat 3.5 g Trans Fat 0 g	Saturated Fat 2 g Trans Fat 0 g
Cholesterol 35 mg	**Cholesterol** 0 mg
Sodium 115 mg	**Sodium** 200 mg
Total Carbohydrates 23 g	**Total Carbohydrates** 23 g
Dietary Fiber 0.25 g Sugars 14 g	Dietary Fiber < 1 g Sugars 12 g
Protein 3 g	**Protein** 1 g

The boxed mix specifies a serving size to be thirty-one grams of dry mix. It's safe to assume the recipe calls for a standard tin used for baking. Can you visualize the size difference between the first and second muffin?

Notice (if you haven't yet) the muffin from the convenience store contains three servings. You would have to slice the muffin in three equal parts to get one portion. Now can you visualize the size difference between the two? Which one is larger, or are they about the same?

If you eat the entire convenience-store muffin, thinking it's one serving and 200 calories, this is what you'll actually consume: 600 calories, 69 grams of processed carbohydrates, and 42 grams of sugar (more on this below). Be certain to read all the relevant information on the label, so you know what you consume.

The store-bought muffin has 50% fat (300/600), and the muffin mix has 25% fat (30/120).

But let's look more closely at the sugar. The store-bought muffin has 14 grams of sugar per serving, which (divided by 4 grams per sugar cube) equals nearly 4 sugar cubes in only one third of a muffin. The whole thing contains 42 grams (14 x 3). Here's the formula:

$$\frac{42 \text{ g of sugar per serving}}{4 \text{ g per sugar cube}} = 10.5 \text{ sugar cubes}$$

In comparison, the muffin mix has 12 grams which is the equivalent of 3 cubes of sugar.

$$\frac{12 \text{ g of sugar per serving}}{4 \text{ g per sugar cube}} = 3 \text{ sugar cubes}$$

By reading nutrition labels, you'll not only get information on the calories, protein, fat, and carbohydrates. You'll also learn what that company deems as one serving.

Manufacturers have the freedom to manipulate serving sizes to make their products seem more attractive to the consumer. This is a common theme with just about any type of food. In fact, we just saw this same thing with the non-dairy creamer. These manufacturers know if you read this label and see "1 muffin = 1 serving = 600 calories," you would probably buy something else.

How many people do you think will pick up this muffin and turn it over to read the nutrition label? Probably not many. If they just glanced at the calories, they'd probably assume the 200 calories listed is for the whole thing, and they may base their purchase on that information.

CONCLUSION

If you purchased the prepackaged muffin, would *you* eat the whole thing? Or would you slice it apart to get your single portion?

Before I changed my lifestyle, I had eaten the whole muffin on several occasions before I began noticing labels (and they were good, good, good!). You can imagine how shocked I was to learn I was eating three servings in one. Today, I no longer desire those muffins, because I know the truth. I also know I would want to eat the entire pastry and wouldn't slice that silly thing into thirds. Instead, I look for healthier alternatives or bring my food with me so I'm not at the mercy of what a store has to offer.

You can't rely on or trust manufacturers to protect your health or interests. They're too busy protecting their own. This is *your* responsibility—no one else's. It is up to you to read those labels thoroughly so you know exactly what you are consuming. If you do, you'll gain insight into why you are or are not getting the results you want with your weight-loss.

Read labels thoroughly, so that you know exactly what you are consuming.

KETCHUP[xliv] *VS.* SPAGHETTI SAUCE[xlv]

Ketchup		Spaghetti Sauce, Traditional	
Serving Size: 1 T (14 g)		Serving Size: ½ cup, 4 oz (112 g)	
Amount Per Serving		Amount Per Serving	
Calories 20 Calories From Fat 0		**Calories** 80 Calories From Fat 18	
Total Fat	0 g	**Total Fat**	2 g
Saturated Fat 0 g Trans Fat 0 g		Saturated Fat 0 g Trans Fat 0 g	
Cholesterol	0 mg	**Cholesterol**	0 mg
Sodium	158 mg	**Sodium**	480 mg
Total Carbohydrates	5 g	**Total Carbohydrates**	13 g
Dietary Fiber 0 g Sugars 4 g		Dietary Fiber 2 g Sugars 8 g	
Protein	0 g	**Protein**	2 g

For dinner, suppose you are cooking turkey in tomato sauce and have these two choices. Let's first compare similar amounts.

Since you are more likely to use ½ cup (spaghetti sauce serving size) with the ground turkey than a tablespoon (ketchup serving size), let's see what the quantities are for ½ cup of ketchup.

There are eight tablespoons in ½ cup. Multiply the ketchup quantities by eight to get comparable nutrition values:

½ cup Serving	Ketchup	Spaghetti Sauce
Total Calories	160 (20 calories x 8 tbsp)	80
Fat (in %)	0	23
Sodium	1264 mg (158 mg x 8 tbsp)	480 mg
Sugar	32/4 = 8 cubes	8/4 = 2 cubes

Ketchup Ingredients: *Tomato concentrate from red ripe tomatoes, distilled vinegar, high-fructose corn syrup, corn syrup, salt, spice, onion powder, natural flavoring.*

Spaghetti Sauce Ingredients: *Tomato Puree (Water, Tomato Paste), Soybean Oil, Salt, Sugar, Dehydrated Onions, Extra Virgin Olive Oil, Spices, Romano Cheese Made From Cow's Milk (Cultured Part-Skim Milk, Salt, Enzymes), Natural Flavors.*

CONCLUSION

Before doing this analysis, I didn't think ketchup was that bad. I certainly was wrong. Now I don't think this is even worthy of being in my home!

If you prefer ketchup and aren't ready to make a drastic change, there are alternatives for you, similar to the bread example earlier.

You may try a lower sodium or lower sugar version. There are also companies that make ketchup with no high-fructose corn syrup. You might even make your own. My mother used to make ours. How times have changed!

The nutritional absolutes you determined earlier will make your decision-making now easier. If you need to keep your sodium low or if you want to rid your diet of high fructose corn syrup, the ketchup would be a bad choice.

PROTEIN SHAKE[xlvi] *VS.* PROTEIN BAR[xlvii]

Protein Shake		Protein Bar	
Serving Size: 1 shake (17 oz)		Serving Size: 1 bar (72g)	
Amount Per Serving		Amount Per Serving	
Calories 280 Calories From Fat 80		**Calories** 270 Calories From Fat 60	
Total Fat	9 g	**Total Fat**	7 g
Saturated Fat 1 g Trans Fat 0 g		Saturated Fat 3 g Trans Fat 0 g	
Cholesterol	25 mg	**Cholesterol**	< 5 mg
Sodium	600 mg	**Sodium**	150 mg
Total Carbohydrates	9 g	**Total Carbohydrates**	32 g
Dietary Fiber 5 g Sugars 0 g		Dietary Fiber 14 g Sugars 3 g	
Protein	40 g	**Protein**	20 g

The fat percentages for the shake and bar are 28% and 22%, respectively. There is minimal sugar in both. So far, so good. But look at the sodium: 600 mg for the drink! I did a double-take when I saw that one.

Which product is right for you?[xlviii] *Neither* may be the right choice. What about your lifestyle? Would something like this help you reach your goals and facilitate weight loss? Are you always on the run and the only way you will get nutrition is by drinking these shakes? Do you insist that more protein helps you get leaner? Whatever you decide, be aware of what's going into your body. Everyone has their own bio-individuality and therefore needs to learn what works best for them.

CONCLUSION

Meal replacement shakes and bars are convenient for people on-the-go or for those who want a quick nutritious meal but don't have time to prepare anything. They tend to be more expensive than natural food. It's easy to get lazy with meal supplements since no preparation is involved, so if you do consume them, remember:

There is no substitute for eating real food for our calories. . This is the best option for success in weight loss and maintenance, so try to limit these meal replacements to no more than one per day.

BUTTER[xlix] *VS.* NON-STICK SPRAY[l]

Butter, salted		Non-Stick Spray	
Serving Size: 1 T (14 g)		Serving Size: About 1/3 Second Spray (.266 g)	
Amount Per Serving		Amount Per Serving	
Calories 100 Calories From Fat 100		**Calories** 0 Calories From Fat 0	
Total Fat	11 g	**Total Fat**	0 g
Saturated Fat 7 g Trans Fat 0 g		Saturated Fat 0 g Trans Fat 0 g	
Cholesterol	30 mg	**Cholesterol**	0 mg
Sodium	90 mg	**Sodium**	0 mg
Total Carbohydrates	0 g	**Total Carbohydrates**	0 g
Dietary Fiber Sugars		Dietary Fiber Sugars	
Protein	0 g	**Protein**	0 g

It seems a little silly to have this comparison, but I want to draw your attention to something.

Butter is 100% fat—that's not news to anyone. But what you might not realize is the non-stick spray is also nearly 100% fat.

Following are the ingredients on the label:

Non-stick Spray Ingredients: *Canola oil*, grain alcohol from corn*

(added for clarity), lecithin from soybeans (prevents sticking), and propellant.
**Adds a trivial amount of fat.*

Notice the calories per serving = 0 on the non-stick spray. Do you know how the manufacturer can state that there are no calories per serving, yet the product is nearly 100% fat?

The serving size states, "About 1/3 of a second of a spray." This is so ridiculous I'm embarrassed for the manufacturer. Do you stand there with a stopwatch and spray for 0.333 seconds? How much time do you actually take to spray your pan?

Oh, and by the way, the manufacturer mentions elsewhere that a 1-second spray covers a 10" skillet. That should be the true serving size. Do you want to guess why it's not? Because if the serving was three times what is listed, there might actually be numbers on the label instead of zeros. Then the company couldn't claim their product is fat free on the front of the bottle.

Furthermore, this manufacturer states in very large letters on the front of the label, "ALL NATURAL." I didn't know propellant was natural. Here is Wikipedia's definition of the word: "A propellant or propellent is a *chemical substance* used in the production of energy or pressurized gas that is subsequently used to create movement of a fluid or to generate propulsion of a vehicle, projectile, or other object" (emphasis mine).

CONCLUSION

Non-stick sprays are great. I use them all the time. But don't be deceived into thinking that there is no fat in this product. It isn't a "freebie," and if you use unlimited amounts, you are probably consuming more fat than you think.

WHOLE EGG[li] *VS.* EGG WHITE[lii]

Whole Egg, Large		Egg White, Large	
Calories 78		Calories 17	
Calories From Fat 45		Calories From Fat 1	
Total Fat	5 g	**Total Fat**	0.1 g
Saturated Fat 1.6 g		Saturated Fat 0 g	
Cholesterol	187 mg	**Cholesterol**	0 mg
Sodium	62 mg	**Sodium**	55 mg
Total Carbohydrates	0.6 g	**Total Carbohydrates**	0.2 g
Dietary Fiber 0 g		Dietary Fiber 0 g	
Sugars 0.6 g		Sugars 0.2 g	
Protein	6 g	**Protein**	3.6 g

As you can see from these labels, the yolk has most of the calories in an egg, all the cholesterol, and nearly all the fat. However, the white has the majority of the protein. The yolk has most of the vitamins and minerals.

CONCLUSION

If you eat only egg whites, you'll consume greater amounts of protein with no fat. You may choose to eat a combination of whole eggs and egg whites, no yolks at all, or have whole eggs all the time.

Egg whites can be purchased as a pre-packaged product. You could also buy several dozen eggs and separate them as you eat them.

If you separate the yolks, what do you do with them? I hate wasting food, so once I tried massaging them on my hair and found it too gross. Now, I cook, cool, and feed them to the stray cats living on my patio. They love them.

STRAWBERRY LOWFAT[liii] VS. PLAIN NONFAT YOGURT[liv]

Strawberry Low Fat Yogurt		Plain Nonfat Yogurt	
Serving Size: 6 oz (170 g)		Serving Size: 1 cup (227 g)	
Amount Per Serving		Amount Per Serving	
Calories 170 Calories From Fat 15		**Calories** 137 Calories From Fat 4	
Total Fat	1.5 g	**Total Fat**	0.4 g
Saturated Fat 1 g Trans Fat 0 g		Saturated Fat 0.3 g Trans Fat	
Cholesterol	10 mg	**Cholesterol**	5 mg
Sodium	85 mg	**Sodium**	189 mg
Total Carbohydrates	33 g	**Total Carbohydrates**	19 g
Dietary Fiber Sugars 26 g		Dietary Fiber 0 g Sugars 19 g	
Protein	5 g	**Protein**	14 g

By now you know what the best decisions are to maximize your weight-loss goals, but just for fun, let's check out the differences on these yogurts.

The biggest difference between the two yogurts is in the sugar, with the low-fat version containing six and one half sugar cubes (26/4 = 6.5). Lactose is a sugar naturally occurring in milk, so this is why there are carbohydrates in both products.

The first example is six ounces, and the second is eight. So with the plain yogurt, you'll have fewer calories and feel fuller longer. Your insulin won't spike, and you will be less likely to crave something later.

CONCLUSION

If you're like me and must have sweetened yogurt, try sprinkling cinnamon over it with some raw trail mix. You may consume a few more calories this way, but you'll derive more nutritional benefit than a sugar-laden option. I also mix in a tablespoon of powdered peanut butter sometimes. You could add nuts to that for texture.

RAISINS[lv] *VS.* FRESH BANANA[lvi]

Raisins		Banana	
Serving Size: 1 small box (43 g)		Serving Size: 1 medium, 7-8" long (118 g)	
Amount Per Serving		Amount Per Serving	
Calories 129 Calories From Fat 2		**Calories** 105 Calories From Fat 4	
Total Fat	0.2 g	**Total Fat**	0.4 g
Saturated Fat 0 g Trans Fat 0 g		Saturated Fat 0.1 g Trans Fat 0 g	
Cholesterol	0 mg	**Cholesterol**	0 mg
Sodium	5 mg	**Sodium**	1 mg
Total Carbohydrates	34 g	**Total Carbohydrates**	27 g
Dietary Fiber 2 g Sugars 25 g		Dietary Fiber 3 g Sugars 14 g	
Protein	1 g	**Protein**	1 g

For this comparison, most values are roughly the same except for the sugar. Notice the 25 grams for the raisins and 14 grams for the banana.

One thing to mention regarding any type of dried fruit is that here fructose is naturally occurring, so its concentration is much higher than fresh fruit, even with a small amount consumed. This isn't a bad thing, but you need to be aware of how your body may respond to high concentrations of simple sugars, regardless of the type.

A second point is in regard to volume. Most of the moisture has been removed from the dried fruit, and a very small portion makes one serving. This may not be enough to satisfy you, and you may wind up eating more than you need. Your best choice might be to eat the fresh banana (almost three times the volume). That way, you consume the roughage or fiber, which will make you fuller and more satisfied sooner. That makes your digestive tract happier too.

CONCLUSION

I have a history of sensitivity to sugar, as I'm sure many of you do. Many relapses could have been avoided if I had been more aware of the impact the foods I ate had on my body. If I had made different choices before putting anything in my mouth, I would not have struggled for as long as I did with the food.

Don't confuse natural fructose with high-fructose corn syrup. These are two different things. We looked at the first one above, so now let's get information about the other.

High-fructose corn syrup[lvii] is made from corn. Cornstarch is processed to yield a type of glucose, which is then processed with enzymes to reach a high percentage of fructose—producing a crystal clear syrup with a much-extended shelf life over sugar. It is also far cheaper to use than real sugar. Now do you see why manufacturers are putting this substance in so many foods? Their motive is cost-savings, not your health.

There is ongoing debate as to the health implications of consuming high-fructose corn syrup. Obviously, we ultimately decide what we eat. I encourage you to do more research on this subject and make informed choices. Reading nutrition labels for the rest of your life will be required for you to stay informed to make the best decisions, for your weight and your health.

Most dried fruit is dehydrated with no additives. However, there will be some versions that have oil or sugar, so always be sure to look at the ingredients.

Also, don't be fooled to think buying something in the health food section of the grocery store means that item is healthy. Always do your homework. Read labels, compare products, and make the wiser choice. Sometimes the best selection is not to buy any at all.

SUMMARY

There are two calculations you need to memorize. The first is for fat:

$$\frac{\textbf{Fat calories per serving}}{\textbf{Total calories per serving}} = \text{\% Fat}$$

The second calculation you need to memorize is for sugar:

$$\frac{\textbf{Sugar grams per serving}}{\textbf{4 grams per sugar cube}} = \text{\# Sugar Cubes}$$

Relying on the front label of any product is not a good idea. Don't be fooled by warm and fuzzy names on the front labels of food items, like "all natural," "homemade," "Granny's oven-baked goodies," "whole wheat," "lite," or "lean." The final word on all packaged food is that shown on the nutrition label and in the ingredient listing.

Ingredients are listed in order, from most occurring to least. If a product lists corn syrup first, that product is mostly sugar, even if it is masquerading as bread, cereal, non-dairy creamer, or something else.

Look at *all* the ingredients on a label to be sure what you are eating. In some products, I have found up to six different kinds of sugar (glucose, fructose, high-fructose corn syrup, molasses, brown or turbinado, and sucrose). These are a few names manufacturers use as a disguise. If these six culprits were all listed as one item, I am certain that sugar would be closer to the top of the ingredient list.

When you first begin your exploration on labels, budget additional time to do the research of products you plan to buy. Bring your calculator, a pencil, and this book or your notes to the grocery store. Take notes right here, on these pages. Cut out labels or take pictures. Tape or staple them into the book, or accumulate a collection of images on your phone for reference.

Making your food at home is a great way to add control over your diet. Download and collect different recipes you are likely to use, and include them here. Use them as your guide.

I love homemade bran muffins. They provide a quick, high-fiber, healthy breakfast for me during those busy mornings. I tried a number of recipes, most of which I didn't like for one reason or another. I substituted applesauce for oil, used a small amount of blackstrap molasses instead of sugar, mixed in whole wheat instead of all-purpose flour, added old-fashioned oats, and cracked in more eggs for protein. Today, I bake these using a recipe I've created from all these substitutions, based on my dietary preferences. I save time not having to read a recipe anymore to make them.

Some of us used to eat all sorts of things, but as we started reading labels, we got pickier and pickier. I hope you do too.

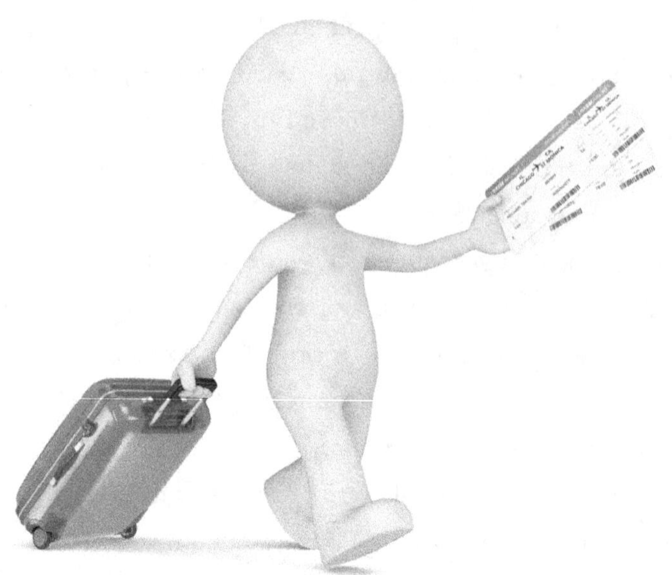

19. FOOD VACATIONS

"I like a little rebellion now and then. It is like a storm in the atmosphere."
—Thomas Jefferson

I was sitting on the floor of a hotel room at 4:00 a.m. with my coffee, pen, hotel stationery, and paper napkins to write on. It was our twelfth wedding anniversary that weekend, and we decided to get away for several days.

My husband and daughter were asleep, but I couldn't keep my eyes closed. I kept thinking about how travel impacts our food plans and wanted to share with you some of these thoughts.

As we were sitting in the restaurant the night before returning home, my husband said, "It will be good to get back to our normal eating routine tomorrow." I agreed.

We all need balance in our lives. Weekends, short trips, and extended vacations are wonderful times to relax and "go with the flow." They are also opportunities to ease up on ourselves.

However, during these times, we don't have as much control over our food choices and have more freedom to relax our diets. This can be to our detriment if we aren't prepared. We can come home feeling angry and depressed, rather than rested and refreshed.

The purpose of a food vacation is to relax our eating program for a specified time. If we plan on and take advantage of these breaks, we will be prepared to enjoy ourselves and will return home re-motivated.

HOW TO PREPARE FOR A FOOD VACATION

"Good instincts usually tell you what to do long before your head has figured it out."
—Michael Burke

Food vacations are exactly what they sound like: a break from the normal routine of our diet plan or formula. As you develop your respites, they will become a part of your program. This may seem counter-intuitive to you right now, but bear with me. Read on and learn about this beautiful balance that you can give yourself.

Planned breaks in your food routine are not for the weak-willed. If you are just starting on your journey, I recommend going one full year before experimenting with a food vacation. Why this long? Because you will have taken your new lifestyle through all the events, ebbs and flows, holidays, and a few unexpected things thrown in.

There's something significant about getting through the first year, since you have worked through all these challenges—and more. This experience will plant your feet firmly on your new path and give you the confidence you need to move to the next level. However, for the first year, be gentle and easy with yourself. Take many precautions to protect yourself, and don't venture too far into unknown territory. There are so many changes to address. The Lord knows that alone will be enough of a challenge to maintain your formula with all the normal stuff going on.

Once your diet and exercise program is fairly well established, I recommend three intentional and well-thought-out breaks from your normal routine:

- Weekends
- Three or four days away from home
- Extended vacations of a week or longer

WEEKEND SPLURGES

Many of us will go off our diets and splurge over the weekends. That's perfectly okay!

Be aware, though, if you want to lose weight and reach your goals, going off your diet at any time will slow your progress. As long as you know this and can get back on track the following Monday, you'll be okay.

Once we do reach our goals, however, a weekend of splurging might not hurt so much. But don't confuse a "binge" with a "splurge." There's a big difference between the two. A binge is an uncontrollable compulsion to keep eating or an inability to stop long after we should have. A splurge is just that—a food vacation over a limited period of time. When Monday comes, we'll get back on track with our diets.

What do you consider to be a splurge? A decadent dessert, a Tex-Mex meal, or a glass of wine or two? If you do splurge, will it trigger a full-fledged binge? Are you lying to yourself by thinking this one time won't hurt? Can you realistically get back on track the following Monday? If not, will this be the beginning of the end of another attempt—and another failure? If you are honest with yourself, do you admit you need to be stricter with your diet on the weekends—for now?

If this is you, then plan ahead. Avoid tempting situations. Some examples could be:

- Attend few or no social activities where food is involved
- Avoid emotionally charged situations, such as family

gatherings

- Make time for yourself each day to meditate and exercise
- Schedule weekly chats with a trusted friend
- Get plenty of rest
- Stay within your financial budget.

Now, why do you think I added the last two points above? If you get too tired, your willpower decreases. It is imperative you take good care of yourself in all ways so your motivation stays strong.

The second point is equally important. If you overspend, you might go into debt. Owing money and having increased monthly payments is stressful. Look at studies online at the havoc this wreaks on individuals and marriages. Don't allow yourself a little fun today at the expense of your long-term weight loss goals. The price is too high.

When I was in high school, I used to look at the thin girls with admiration. As we ate lunch in the cafeteria, I would study what and how they ate. I tried to duplicate what I saw by bringing similar portion sizes in my lunch bag. These girls seemed to peck at their food, without really devouring it (which is something I did well). Others wouldn't even eat—perhaps they only ate one meal a day, but they were rail-thin.

I failed miserably trying to eat like thin people. I simply couldn't do it. Many years later, I realized I wasn't taking the appropriate steps to eat like a normal person. I wasn't starting where I stood at that moment. Instead, I was projecting to where I wanted to be and trying to control the outcome.

Obviously, I was obsessed with food in more ways than one. The mental preoccupation had to be addressed. I had to get on a nutritionally sound diet. I needed direction from someone. I needed structure by spacing my meals apart—not too close together, yet not too far apart, either. In trying to mimic someone else's program, I was doomed to fail.

This is a mistake I see people often make—they begin their formula where they want to be, rather than where they are at that moment. For example, you might want to eat like a person who weighs fifty pounds less than you. If you did that, you would mess up your body and your mind. Without a doubt, you would relapse and give up.

You must begin your program exactly where you are today. Begin with YOU in the beginning, and no one else.

What are you currently eating? What times of day do you usually eat? How many meals do you consume each day, and what quantities? These are the numbers to begin with.

If you currently eat a mostly fast food diet, begin by substituting one meal with more healthful choices (nutrition). If you prefer late night meals, try to take them a bit earlier for a change (metabolism). If you skip breakfast, begin your day with a small thing, such as a cup of yogurt (metabolism). If your meals are too large, then decrease the quantity by using a smaller plate (calories).

This is your life and these are your decisions. Change one thing at a time. This process is slower, but it is more certain. It will also establish a lifetime of good habits.

THREE OR FOUR DAYS AWAY FROM HOME

Are you flying or driving? Will you be at a hotel, and will you have access to a refrigerator, stove, oven, or microwave? All this information will help you plan to maintain your program so you keep eating your familiar foods—at least some of the time.

If you want to carry some of your food with you, decide approximately how many meals you will eat out each day. From that point, determine how much food you may need to bring. For example, if I know I will be eating one restaurant meal per day (lunch or dinner), I'll need to bring breakfasts, snacks, and other non-perishable food for the rest of that day. Keep in mind, however, that restaurant meals can be heavier and more calorie-dense, so you may not need to take as much food as you first thought.

It's best to bring more items from home, rather than fewer, even if they're not eaten. You can always take the excess home.

What do I mean by this? Well, you can bring one snack for each day. Toss in a full-sized box (new and sealed is best) of your healthy cereal, a plastic bowl and spoon, and when you arrive, buy a quart of skim milk to keep in the mini-fridge or ice chest.

Also, consider bringing a variety of other healthy items you eat most days. Rice cakes and peanut butter tubs are great (if you are okay with the latter); cans of tuna fish and an opener; and a large, portable, refillable water bottle to stay hydrated and keep your physiology in top shape. Don't forget your vitamins and medications.

Think about any daily food-related habit that you are able to maintain with a little forethought, and bring it on your trip. Be sure to multiply those items by the number of days you'll be gone.

One time I was packing for a long trip, and. I put a can of whey protein in my suitcase. It had already been opened, so it wasn't a new, safety-sealed container. I had a powdery surprise when I opened my suitcase! It was all over everything. Today, if there's a risk of this happening, I'll place the item in a plastic bag. I may even double-bag it.

Another time, I wanted to take hardboiled eggs. I placed about a dozen in a plastic bag. I thought leaving them in the shell would protect them even more.

When I arrived at the hotel room, I opened my suitcase. I had a mixed, mushy bag of shell bits, egg yolks, and egg white. Yuck!

EXTENDED VACATIONS

Surprisingly, these trips may be the easiest to stay on track, since you can develop a stable routine over a longer time period. Where you stay has so much to do with your ability to stick to your formula. Get all the information you need before your trip so you can prepare well. Here are some thoughts to consider before you leave:

- Is there a small refrigerator in the room, or can you have one delivered for a small fee?

- If you bring an ice chest, you'll need to replenish the ice each day and drain the water. Is there an ice machine on the hotel floor?

- Will there be a coffee pot and supplies in the room? Do you need to bring additional cream, sweetener, etc.?

- Look online at menus from the hotel restaurant and those nearby. Decide in advance what to eat and what to avoid.

- Is there a sundry or convenience store on the hotel grounds?

- Is there a traditional grocery store nearby?

It is unrealistic to think you will keep a squeaky-clean diet on an extended vacation. What I suggest is to try to maintain your current weight. Don't put pressure on yourself to lose weight during a vacation. Just have fun, and if you do happen to lose weight, consider that an added bonus.

Another thing you can do is be more physically active to temporarily compensate for the indulgences of the diet. I wouldn't recommend this type of compensation on a normal basis. It only leads to trouble and disappointment.

You may not feel so great upon your return, carrying a few more pounds, but what you will likely gain is a renewed motivation to begin your formula once again. I have become so disgusted with myself during some food vacations when I've strayed far from my diet, I can't *wait* to get back home for some clean eating!

SUMMARY

It may seem contradictory to have a food vacation and plan to eat your normal diet at the same time. But the longer the vacation, the more normal food you should bring, not only because of the length of the stay, but also because of your physiology.

Here's why: your body chemistry can get thrown off from eating differently from your normal routine. The longer you eat high-calorie or unusual foods, the harder it will be to get back on track when you return home. This is because your chemistry has been altered by the additional fat, sugar, salt, additives, and processed carbohydrates consumed away from home.

The action of taking your normally eaten food along is like purchasing an insurance policy. You want to do the risky thing (eating fun food), but you also want to re-stabilize your chemistry when you return (eating normally again).

Taking your low-calorie edibles on a food vacation works to insure that you will get back on track upon your return. It signifies a future intention.

The main point to remember with the food vacation is that it is for a limited time and for the purpose of "resting" from your normal regime. This healthy practice can increase the quality of your life.

Once again, the farther you get off track during a food vacation, the harder you will have to work to get back on track when you return home.

Try to adhere somewhat to your successful diet plan, and don't let yourself go completely. When you return home, give yourself time to re-adjust, and take it easy if/when you struggle. If you persist in your efforts, you will experience a new sense of motivation and determination to succeed with your weight-loss goals.

SECTION II:
FORMULA BUSTERS

"A successful man is one who can lay a firm foundation with the bricks others have thrown at him." —David Brinkley

Formula Busters are behaviors, responses, habits, or events that can interfere with or prevent you from reaching your weight-loss goals. After each of these pitfalls, I have also listed an accompanying "Formula Factor," which is a healthy response you can take to counter it.

Your basic personality determines much of how you respond to life. Some of you, like me, are highly-strung, and everything seems to bug you. Others of you may be laid-back and rarely get flustered—or you may be somewhere in between.

When things throw you off—and they will—your response is vital to success with your food program. A wise person has said, "What happens to you is less important than how you respond to it."

There are two things to consider. The first is what your natural tendencies are. How do you typically react in stressful situations? Do you turn to food for comfort?

The second is how you choose to respond despite your negative emotions. Do you fly off the handle and react, or think about the problem and calmly respond? If you know you have given in to unhealthy reactions in the past toward unpleasant people or events, how can you change this? Can you list specifically what you would like to do differently? Finally, will you take these items to your morning quiet time and ask God to help you overcome your unhealthy reactions?

If you aren't reaching your goals, a Formula Buster or two might be sabotaging your efforts. Your job is to discover what these are. After that, you need to experiment with modes of thought or behavior that are deliberately different.

Utilizing as many Formula Factors as possible protects you from failure. The more solution-conscious we become, the more likely we will succeed with our weight-loss goals.

FORMULA BUSTER #1: SPONTANEOUS EATING

"I adore spontaneity, providing it is carefully planned." —Unknown

Spontaneous eating can take many forms and may include sampling at the grocery store or mall food court, nibbling from a co-worker's candy jar, eating leftover Halloween candy, or munching on the bread or chips a restaurant serves upon your arrival. Other saboteurs might be food "gifts" or birthday parties for you or the staff at the office, the cute kid down the street asking you to support his school by buying a chocolate bar, or a table of Girl Scout cookies for sale outside the grocery store.

I have sometimes asked these fund-raiser kids if I can merely write a check. They have always said, "No, you have to buy something. We can't take donations like that." I have rarely been able to donate money to these organizations without receiving the junk I really don't want. So today, I may only buy one and give it to someone who wants it—or I may not support the organization at all. But I absolutely will not sabotage myself with bringing tempting junk food into my house!

HEIDI'S STORY

Heidi is a young, single, professional woman. She has a high-stress job, works late most nights, eats a nutritionally imbalanced diet, and doesn't budget time to work out.

Most days, Heidi gets to the office early and skips her breakfast because she feels it's a hassle and there's no time to eat it. She has no appetite in the morning anyway, so this is justifiable in her mind.

When she arrives at the office, there are usually several dozen hot, fresh doughnuts on the conference room table. All of a sudden, she's hungry, so she grabs one, wolfs it down, and returns to work.

Soon, her mind starts obsessing about another doughnut. Finding some papers she needs to copy, she heads to the Xerox. Although a machine is next to her office, she goes to the one near the conference room at the other side of the building. She discretely scopes out the hall. No one's around. She slips into the conference room to get a second doughnut and tucks it under the papers, returning to her office without making the copies. She hides it in her desk and sneaks bites, careful to make sure no one notices.

A little while later, she starts thinking about the doughnuts again and decides to speak with a co-worker whose office is (surprise!) near the conference room. She picks up another doughnut after her conversation and returns to her office. This pattern repeats until she has consumed four doughnuts by lunchtime.

Of course, then she's not really hungry, so at 3:00 p.m., she buys a diet soda and a candy bar from the vending machine. She eats nothing else and works until 6:00 p.m.

When she gets home, she devours some chips while waiting for her instant mac-and-cheese to heat in the microwave. For dessert, the remains of a gallon of butter pecan ice cream await her in the freezer.

Heidi wakes up the next morning without an appetite and begins the process again.

At her annual appointment with her gynecologist, she was found to have added forty pounds over the last year. She knew she had put on weight, but the realization shocked her. At the same time, she also felt a sense of relief. She was now prepared for change.

She asked her doctor to refer her to a nutritionist, and she also started seeing a life coach to begin the process of changing her habits.

QUESTION

When Heidi realized she had put on so much weight, she was shocked. This is understandable. But why do you suppose she was relieved? Jot down your thoughts on paper, and we'll come back to this question later.

FORMULA FACTOR: STRUCTURED EATING

Heidi learned from the nutritionist to plan her weekly meals and stock her kitchen with healthy foods. She needed to take time to prepare her food in advance. When arriving home from work, she only had to heat that day's evening meal and eat a salad while she waited. Breakfast, meals, and snacks every day became a necessity, not an option. She purchased a small cooler to hold everything and took it with her to work.

She also started walking five days a week. Exercising developed a healthier lifestyle and helped her lose the weight faster.

From the life coach, Heidi gained invaluable help. She learned tools to handle her stress without abusing food. She gained insight into herself that made her a stronger individual.

After a year, Heidi felt comfortable enough to end her relationship with the nutritionist, but she kept seeing the life coach on a more limited basis to help her cope with ups and downs.

To curb Heidi's habit of sampling in grocery stores, she learned to eat a small snack before shopping. This gave her more willpower to say no.

Now, back to the question as to why Heidi was relieved: because she had finally reached the point where reality and her willingness to change coincided. The game was over, and it was time to get to work on her health.

Did you guess right? Of more importance, have *you* reached the place where you are so sick and tired of losing the food-battle, you are willing to change? What are you going to do about it?

FORMULA BUSTER #2: NO PORTION CONTROL

"But the fruit of the Spirit is love, joy, peace, patience, kindness, goodness, faithfulness, gentleness, and self-control. Against such things there is no law."
—Galatians 5:22-23

Many of us know a portion of protein should be no larger than a deck of cards, a serving of fruit or vegetables the size of a baseball, and carbohydrates no more than a standard light bulb.[lviii]

Before we realize it, the card deck has become super-sized, the baseball a softball, and the light bulb a floodlight. Our mind plays funny tricks on us.

STEVE'S STORY

Steve isn't happy with his body, but he feels trapped in his lifestyle. An outside salesman, he is overweight, inactive, and on the road frequently.

On an ordinary day, Steve wakes and sorts through his e-mails for an hour or two with a cup of coffee. Then he gets in the car to call on customers for the rest of the day. He never thinks about planning meals or taking them with him. After an hour, he stops for gas at his usual convenience store with a fast-food restaurant inside. It's lunchtime by now, and he's hungry. He grabs his favorite on-the-road meal: a double-meat bacon cheeseburger, jumbo fries, and large soda.

In the evening, Steve's energy is sapped, so he orders a 16-inch delivery pizza and a large soft drink, and eats while he finishes his work. Every day, this cycle repeats itself.

The turning point for Steve occurred when he attended his twin brother's wedding. He had a great time with all the festivities, but he came home feeling depressed and aware of the emptiness of his life. He wanted to stop his crazy eating, attract a pretty girl, and get married like his brother. He also realized the lack of an eating structure in his life would play havoc with his health.

Steve wanted to feel good physically and have energy, and he knew exercise needed to be a part of his life. Mostly, he knew that if he kept up his present lifestyle, his chances of achieving any of these ideals were almost nil.

He liked his job and wanted to maintain his current work schedule, so he took a course at the community college on healthy eating habits. He searched online for creative ways to work out while working away from home. Based on the resource's recommendations, he purchased some home equipment at a local fitness store. He began a realistic exercise program of three to four times a week at home or in a hotel.

FORMULA FACTOR: PORTION CONTROL

After finishing his course on eating habits, Steve understood more specifically what he was doing wrong with his food and what he needed to change:

- Nutritional content
- Portion control
- Meal frequency

He realized that it had been convenient for him to have only one or two meals a day, since eating was a hassle to him.

The first thing Steve changed was his decision to eat breakfast at home every morning before he got on the road. He bought several healthy breakfast choices at the grocery store and kept these items available. He committed himself to weekly trips to the grocers so these supplies would stay replenished.

The next changes Steve made were his choices at the mini-mart. Instead of going to the fast food area for his meal, he searched through the limited choices at the store. He found a low-sugar protein drink, a bottle of iced coffee to mix with it, a banana by the register, and a granola bar. He also bought an additional high-protein bar for a snack later before he arrived home. This prevented his getting too hungry before dinner.

One problem Steve encountered, even with making healthier choices, was portion control. If he chose to buy a bag of low-fat chips instead of the granola bar, he found that many of the bags contained several servings. He didn't want to go through the hassle of looking at all those labels, so after doing a bit of detective work, he decided to purchase the same thing every time he visited the store.

On the way home, he wasn't so ravenous because he had eaten better throughout the day. So he took time to stop by a grocery store that made prepared foods. There he ordered a normal portion of a protein, a veggie, and a complex carbohydrate. With a good meal boxed and ready, he came home to enjoy a filling and healthy dinner.

For Steve, a lack of structure with his eating had created his portion control problem. Once he began eating more regularly, he didn't become so hungry, so he didn't want or need all that extra food. Furthermore, because he was making healthier choices throughout the day, he felt better, had more energy to work out, and began losing the weight. He was happy to find himself becoming the person he wanted to be.

I still wrestle with portion control today. I've removed all the junk from my house. I don't buy stuff that tempts me, but many days I want more than I need and feel deprived if I try to overcome my desire.

Here is where the power of prayer can save you and me. Say a prayer right there in the kitchen. Ask God for self-control and for Him to guide you. Tell Him of your intention to reach your goal. Tell Him you are determined to use His power to overcome the enemy.

You already know what a serving size looks like. But here's your real battle. Knowledge won't help you when what you really need is *power*. And through Jesus Christ, we have that power to win the battle.

"But thanks be to God! He gives us the victory through our Lord Jesus Christ." —1 Corinthians 15:57

It's important to focus on God's forgiveness of our mistakes. When we fail, it's easy to fall into self-condemnation. The feeling of self-loathing will set us up for more failure. We have to change our minds before we can change our actions, and prayer is the only thing that will consistently overcome this problem.

"Therefore, I urge you, brothers, in view of God's mercy, to offer your bodies as living sacrifices, holy and pleasing to God—this is your spiritual act of worship. Do not confirm any longer to the pattern of this world, but be transformed by the renewing of your mind." —Romans 12:1-2

FORMULA BUSTER #3: FAT OR FICTION

"Deception may give us what we want for the present, but it will always take it away in the end." —Rachel Hawthorne

If you believe in a lie, does that make it true? If you ignore some part of reality, does that mean it doesn't exist? If you listen to a falsehood enough, it may become truth to you. What are you feeding your mind?

In 2 Corinthians 10:5, Paul says, *"We take captive every thought to make it obedient to Christ."* This includes gathering information about foods you eat. In order to achieve your goals, the sources you depend on must be sound.

How will you know you can rely on the information you receive?"

You first ask and count on God to lead you to people and resources. Trust in Him to do this. Keep praying for wisdom in all things, especially your food choices.

CARMAN'S STORY

Discouragement gripped Carman. After attempting a "low-fat" diet for three months, she had seen few results.

Before starting her diet, Carman ate red meat most nights and drank whole milk each day. She decided that she needed to start paying attention to her food's fat content. She began purchasing products with labels advertising "lean" on chicken, turkey, and beef. She also switched the whole milk for 2%. Her weight didn't change much. What went wrong? She was baffled.

FORMULA FACTOR: HOW MUCH FAT?

Although the label on ground turkey read "lean," she didn't know that the meat packing industry uses that term to mean 10 grams of fat or less per 100 grams of food. However, when she learned to divide the fat calories per serving by the total calories per serving, she discovered the ground turkey contained 41% fat. It was *not* lean meat!

In the same way, the label on ground beef read "90% lean, 10% fat." When Carman applied the same calculation, she discovered the meat was a whopping 53% fat.

The 2% milk also figured to be much higher in fat. When Carman turned the bottle around and read the nutrition label, she found it contained 43% fat.

No wonder Carman was discouraged! She had been using bad information. Once she learned how to read labels and calculate fat calories, she began to choose different products. She began to see results on her scale.

Now she shops with calculator in hand and reads the nutrition labels on the back of the products. This simple calculation has made a marked difference in her food choices:

Fat Calories/Svg ÷ Total Calories/Svg = % Fat

FORMULA BUSTER #4: OFFICE PARTY DISASTERS

"Commit to the Lord whatever you do, and your plans will succeed."
—Proverbs 16:3

Office parties—who invented these things, anyway? Some saboteur, no doubt, whose sole intent was to wreck our healthy eating programs.

You know what to expect. A buffet table filled with high-calorie snacks, chips and dips, a luscious cake in honor of the boss's birthday or the season (Christmas, Mardi Gras, etc.), and a bowl of well-spiked punch.

To say "no" would be rude, so you fill a festive paper plate with a piece of cake and a few snacks. You accept a cup filled with you-know-what. After all, you have to join the toast to the man who signs your paycheck, right? "Cheers!"

The alcohol lowers your inhibitions, and your careful plans fly out the window. As you socialize with your fellow workers, the conversation draws your attention away from your commitment. You suddenly realize you have eaten much of the cake, most of the chips, a handful of nuts, and are reaching for more.

FORMULA FACTOR: OFFICE PARTY SUCCESS

If you arrive at the party and find absolutely no healthy foods to eat, you can make the best of this situation by avoiding all trigger foods. Period. Don't even tempt yourself. Other actions you can take are:

- Remove bread off sandwiches and eat the meat and veggies.

- Eat the fresher-looking foods (the ones with vegetables in them).

- Avoid anything fried.

- Abstain from chips and crackers (trigger foods that encourage unconscious eating).

- Place some food on a plate or napkin, so you appear to be eating.

- Drink coffee, water, or diet soda—keeping the cup or glass in your hand at all times.

- Eat something before you go.

- Approach people you want to know better and show interest in their lives. They won't notice whether you eat or not.

- Smile as if you're having a wonderful time, and you might actually begin to have fun.

- Call a friend before you go. Affirm your commitment to stay on your program. Follow up afterward or ask them to call you to see how you did.

Many office parties take place in early afternoon. The business closes early in honor of So-and-so, and sandwiches or pizzas are ordered. Out come the other offerings—mixed nuts, sour cream dip, crackers and cheese, and the heavily frosted cake. There's no time to disappear and eat a healthy lunch. If you have a cache of food items at your desk, you can sneak a little something beforehand and give yourself more self-control.

If the party takes place in the evening, plan to eat a full meal prior to the party and not eat anything at all there. This may be difficult due to peer pressure, but unless you draw attention to yourself, no one will notice. If you know what will be catered, you have even more control over your choices.

Alternatively, if you want to make this a "food vacation," you will need to sacrifice one of your free days for this one. Just be certain to adhere to your plan.

Warning: It's easy to say you will have a free food day at the party and focus on the diet later. However, with so many of us, what happens is we let the next day—and the next—and the next become free ones also. Be aware of this danger before the party begins, and make a firm decision before you arrive. The important thing is to make a commitment, stick with it, and accept the consequences of your choice.

FORMULA BUSTER #5: RESTAURANT LUNCHES

"God doesn't want people to do what they think is best: he wants them to do what he knows is best, and no amount of reasoning and intellectualizing will discover that." —Henry T. Blackaby

Eating out doesn't have to be a disaster for one's diet, but it does require a tremendous amount of willpower and planning.

Is the food served at a particular restaurant especially tempting for you, or is it easy to make healthy choices there? Can you be the one who decides where to eat? Are you with a friend who supports you in your diet endeavors, or will they unknowingly sabotage your efforts? Finally, how often do you eat at a restaurant? Believe it or not, frequently dining out can and will wear down your defenses.

For me, it's simply not worth it anymore to go out too often. The unaccustomed food makes me feel hung over the next day, as if I were not myself. I have less energy until I get back on track. It's expensive too. Have you ever looked at your receipt and considered how many home-cooked meals you could have purchased for the amount you spent on that one restaurant meal?

FORMULA FACTOR: ADVANCE DECISIONS

You have to decide what's right for you. For me, I average one restaurant meal each week at most. Vacations and holidays are, of course, my exceptions.

Deciding on a restaurant can be the key factor in your success or failure. If you go to the one that serves extra-tempting food, you might make this a free food day instead of agonizing over what you aren't able to eat. If you're able to make healthy choices and still be content, then do so, but it might be easier to go someplace else.

Whom you dine with can also make a difference. Stick with the winners! If you want to be thin, hang around with thin people. Of course, that's not always possible. You may have to entertain a co-worker or a client. In this case, you have several options:

- You can eat something before you go
- Call it a free food day
- Try to make the best choice available

Remember, how often you dine out can play a big part in how fast you lose—or gain—weight. You may not have a choice. The truth is the more frequently you eat at restaurants, the wiser your choices will have to be and the fewer free food days you can take.

FORMULA BUSTER #6: BUSINESS TRIPS

"You will never reach your destination if you stop and throw stones at every dog that barks." —Winston Churchill

If business trips are part of your profession, you will need to learn some tools to help you stay on your program while away from home.

WALTER'S STORY

Walter has an annual four-day convention in another state. He works in his company's booth and rooms with a co-worker. He usually stays in a high-end host hotel that has a workout facility, restaurant, coffee shop, and room service.

Walter hurriedly packed his bag the night before his flight and rushed out of the house the next morning. By the time he neared the gate at the airport, he realized he was hungry. Before the plane loaded, he got a pastry and coffee at the airport kiosk.

The tradeshow hours were long, with candy the only snack in the booth. The crazy pace left hardly any time to use the restroom, let alone get a healthy meal somewhere.

When the tradeshow floor closed each day, Walter stopped by the hotel coffee shop and wolfed down a deli sandwich with chocolate milk. Later, he was expected to meet with potential clients. This meant late nights, heavy restaurant meals, and lots of alcohol.

By the time the convention ended and Walter flew home, he felt horrible from all the junk food, drinking, and late-night eating with customers. He wished he had taken time to plan better for his trip.

He wants to adhere closer to his normal diet/exercise program, but doesn't know how to dovetail his lifestyle with the conventions. These are parts of his profession, so he needs to learn some tools to insure his success while traveling.

If this is your lifestyle as well, you need not fall into the same trap as Walter. A little advance planning will help you stay with your healthy eating program.

FORMULA FACTOR: PLANNING

Check the hotel amenities before traveling. Is there a free breakfast? What do they serve? Is there a copy of the room service menu you could look at? What does the hotel restaurant serve? Is there a fitness room or track nearby? If so, bring workout clothes in case you have an opportunity to exercise. Do they have a small refrigerator in each room, or can one be delivered to the room for the duration of the stay?

Pack non-perishable, lightweight food items to keep in the hotel room. Your luggage will take a beating, so find some that are small, sturdy, and easily stored. Some examples might be protein bars, small vacuum travel packets of tuna or peanut butter, and packages of whole-wheat crackers. If you have a refrigerator in your room, you can find a grocery store nearby and purchase milk for cereal (don't forget the plastic bowl and spoon), and other refrigerated items to help you stay on track.

Bring healthy snacks to the trade show. Carry an insulated bag containing a protein drink, a piece of fruit from the hotel lobby, and a granola bar. Find the lulls in the tradeshow when you can slip to the back of the booth and grab a bite or take a sip. These frequent health-breaks will keep your blood sugar at a normal level.

Discern between mandatory, productive events, and social events that serve little purpose for professional networking. If a dinner is a company meal, it is mandatory and, most likely, productive. But to hook up at the bar and drink all night on the company tab doesn't have as much to do with business or networking as it does with indulgence. It won't do much to rejuvenate you for the next long day, either. Don't just go with the flow. Decide what is important and necessary, and stick with your formula as much as possible.

Communicate with the roommate. Let them know at the beginning of the trip that you will have food in the hotel room and you probably won't stay out late. Setting boundaries at the beginning of the trip helps both parties know what to expect.

FORMULA BUSTER #7: NO EXIT STRATEGY

"A goal without a plan is just a wish." —Antoine de Saint-Exupéry

A lot of folks enroll in rigorous weight-loss programs, intending to eventually adapt the new lifestyle changes into their daily routines. At some point, they realize their efforts have failed. This can happen especially with plans that provide pre-cooked, pre-packaged food. Most will have to go back to cooking their own food and not purchasing all those expensive meals.

Others may embark on a fitness program that requires more commitment than they can fit into their lifestyle. They soon get burned out and drop the entire thing. Perhaps they were too ambitious and their expectations were too high.

To try new approaches and release less favored ones—this is all part of the process of finding your formula. Expect to experience trials and errors along the way. You will grow stronger in the journey.

JOHN'S STORY

John is overweight by thirty-five pounds and does no exercise. He has recently been selected to participate in his local TV station's version of "The Biggest Loser." He will be working with a trainer who will put him on a fitness and diet program for twelve weeks, the duration of the contest.

After the first week, John realizes he doesn't agree with all the trainer is suggesting, but, determined to win this contest, he follows the instructions. He knows his lifestyle up to this point hasn't worked, and that's what has motivated him to participate.

About midway through the contest, John is really excited about his results. At that point, he begins to wonder, "How will I maintain this new lifestyle without my trainer and the scrutiny of the press?"

FORMULA FACTOR: EXIT STRATEGY

John can proactively devise an exit strategy during the contest in anticipation of its imminent conclusion. He realizes he may lose some of the benefits once he is on his own. He likes this program right now, but doesn't want to continue all facets of it for the long run.

How can he dovetail the prescribed exercise and diet with his regular lifestyle in order to maintain his results? What does he want to keep? What can he let go?

He will have to decide which changes he can live with, those he will continue, and those he can modify.

For example, what time of day will he do cardio? The trainer may insist on first thing in the morning. For the duration of the contest, John will follow those instructions. But his exit strategy is for the evening, when he is more comfortable with working out. He will try this for a while to see how it works and readjust the schedule if necessary.

Another example of an exit strategy could be diet modification. The trainer has him on an ultra-high-protein diet. John questions its nutritional soundness, but he stays on the program because he knows it's temporary.

His exit strategy might be to eat smaller portions of protein when the program is over, obtaining other calories from fibrous carbohydrates, starchy ones, and some fats. Again, he will try this for a while to see if he can maintain his weight and if it fits in with his normal life.

FORMULA BUSTER #8: NO ACCOUNTABILITY

"It is not only what we do, but also what we do not do, for which we are accountable." —Moliere

ccountability can mean the difference between success and failure in any venture.

How can you become accountable to someone or something in order to help reach your goals? What or who can make you answerable with the food so that you are driven to do better? Do you call a friend each day to say what you plan to eat? Do you attend a weight-loss support group? Fitness classes and gatherings help many people, but others do not feel comfortable in such settings. How will you find motivation for your fitness?

In order to fully develop your formula, you must find answers to these questions. Humans are stronger while working with others. If left on your own, it is too easy to forget your goals and resume your old habits.

Are you aware of the value of being accountable to someone? Do you see the necessity for accountability when it comes to your food and weight loss goals?

Counselors, personal trainers, nutritionists, life coaches, family, employers, spouses, partners, and friends—the list of supportive people is endless. Nevertheless, if you are going to invest part of your life with someone, or at least share your personal needs with them, approach the relationship with caution and have a goal. Know what you want from that person and what your expectations are, and let them know these things too.

ALISA'S STORY

Alisa wanted to lose twenty pounds, attain a habit of exercising regularly, and develop more personal initiative with her career. She had been trying to motivate herself to do these things for two years and hadn't been successful. She realized she needed help in attaining her goals, and felt that hiring a life coach might be the first step.

A method of accountability was something Alisa felt she lacked. A good coach could help keep her on track and measure her progress in all the areas where she wanted to see growth. Eager to get started, she hired the first life coach she found through an advertisement. During the first session, she was very specific about what she expected.

Unfortunately, things didn't work out as well as she planned. Alisa wanted the coach to probe, to give her introspective assignments in preparation for the next session, to provide her with referrals for diet and exercise, and to be a resource of information and accountability.

Instead, the life coach only encouraged Alisa to buy her products— her books, seminars, and workshops. She addressed almost nothing toward Alisa's needs. "Purchase my materials," she insisted. "They will give you the answers to your problems."

Alisa disagreed and grew suspicious of the woman's motives. She realized she had been too quick to hire someone and had failed to check references or look at reviews. She was so eager to reach for help she didn't see the problems as they developed.

After three months, little to no progress on her goals, and a huge financial loss, she decided to fire the coach and look for a new one.

FORMULA FACTOR: ACCOUNTABILITY

Most people agree we all need to be accountable to someone in our lives. We owe our children our good influence, to set examples for them so they can one day become productive members of society. We need loyalty to our spouse or significant other, to uphold our commitments to them, and treat them with love and respect on a daily basis. We are called to serve our country, to uphold the values our nation was founded on, and to take action where necessary to preserve our freedoms.

We can make ourselves accountable to others by getting involved in a local gym and, in this way, lead by example. We can find a workout partner for strength training. We can go to cycling classes where we meet others and develop relationships. We can join a weight-loss support group and develop friendships while losing those unwanted pounds.

Associating ourselves with people who have similar goals will have a positive effect on us and will deepen our resolve to change our habits.

Everybody has different accountability needs. It is your job to determine yours. Do you need frequent contacts with your sources of support? If so, stay connected, no matter how much progress you've made. You will gain more confidence if you do. If something unexpected happens, you can tap in to your support system for help.

Are you generally self-motivated? Do you only need periodic jump-starts through a session with a personal trainer for fresh ideas? How about a quarterly appointment with a nutritionist for reevaluating your diet plan? Get connected with professionals you trust. Check in with them regularly for refreshment and new ideas.

As you examine yourself honestly, you can determine the level of accountability you need right now. Be open to trying different groups or professionals so you will reach your goals as quickly as possible. Because life is not static, there may be times when you need more or less support, so be sensitive to your needs. Always stay in touch with your feelings. Don't hesitate to reach out.

If you are accountable to a professional (e.g., personal trainer, life coach, or nutritionist) for a limited time, begin this relationship with the expectation that it will be temporary. Come to each session with goals and questions. Get as much out of this time as possible. Think about the many ways you will transition out of this into your normal life, taking along with you some permanent changes. In this way, when the end of the relationship is reached, you will move forward with confidence.

Before hiring anyone, interview people you have an interest in working with. Ask friends and associates for references. Always check online reviews, if available. Know your expectations before interviewing, and communicate these during the first session. If the person isn't responsive to your needs, find another one.

Don't forget to check credentials. For many, connecting with a professional to help them get a jump-start on a program is necessary and helpful. However, get it right the first time, and you will save time and money as you reach your goals.

Remember, these professionals are working for you. You have hired them. You pay them to work for you. You are their boss.

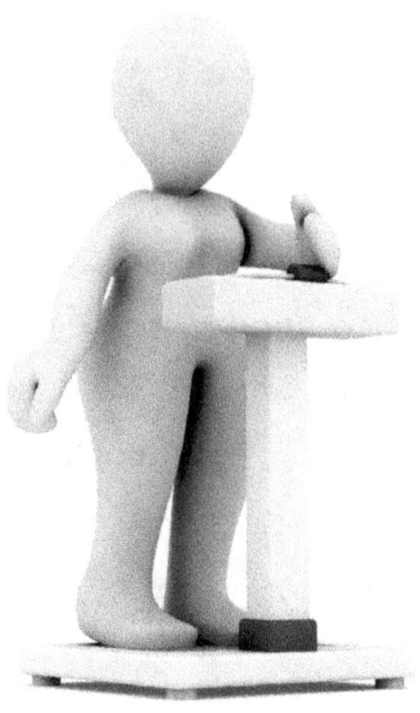

FORMULA BUSTER #9: OBSESSED WITH WEIGHING

"You become what you think about all day long."
—Ralph Waldo Emerson

Are you someone who defines yourself by a number on the scale? Are you fixated on a specific number for your ideal weight? Read on to see how this might work against you.

GINA'S STORY

Gina was in the process of dieting and losing pounds. She stepped on a doctor's scale every morning and kept meticulous records of her meals and weight.

Her trend was a consistent weight loss. Some months she lost more than others, but Gina didn't recognize her success and felt discouraged. Why?

On the days she didn't see a decrease in her weight or when she actually saw an increase, she became depressed and angry. She couldn't focus on her work and avoided talking to people. A pound or two of weight loss didn't translate into better relationships with others or a better quality of life.

On her doctor's advice, she began weighing once a month. This released her from the preoccupation with the scale's numbers. She increased her focus in other areas that brought her more pleasure.

FORMULA FACTOR: NO WEIGH!

You may need to get rid of the scale if it causes you to be obsessed. If you weigh more than once a week, you tend to keep the focus on the weight. This can lead to an unhealthy obsession.

Gauge your weight-loss progress by how your clothes fit and feel on your body. Get in tune with these things and forget the numbers. If you must keep the scale, then only weigh once a week.

I have struggled with defining myself by the number I see on the scale. So today, I rarely weigh. I let the doctors keep those records for me.

FORMULA BUSTER #10: HIDDEN SUGAR

"Human beings have a demonstrated talent for self-deception when their emotions are stirred." —Carl Sagan

We've talked about how manufacturers deceive us with fat and sugar, as well as use deceptive labeling to sell more products. In another section, sugar was determined to be one of the most common trigger foods. Finally, the emotional impact sugar has on one's mind is often an issue with people who struggle with food. The physiological/chemical effect on your brain, coupled with the comfort of association is a double-whammy that keeps many in denial about their weight problem.

Read on for Brenda's story and how she was able to overcome this sneaky substance.

BRENDA'S STORY

Brenda kept failing at her diet, and she couldn't figure out why she was unable to stay with her diet plan.

It wasn't a severely strict diet, either. It eliminated most forms of sugar and processed carbohydrates, but allowed her several "cheats" throughout the week. In addition, it was nutritionally balanced, with sufficient amounts of calories, fat, protein, and carbohydrates.

Brenda loved coffee. She drank two cups every morning. After lunch, she had to have another cup. In the late afternoon, she indulged in several cups of decaf. Her average was five cups a day.

For every cup of coffee, Brenda would pour about one-fourth cup of flavored liquid creamer in her cup. Does that sound like a lot? You may be surprised!

She had a variety of these creamers, depending upon her mood. Although she knew there was some sugar in them, she assumed it couldn't be much. She was never concerned about the impact it might have on her diet. After all, this was an innocuous accessory to her coffee, an essential of her day…

The problem was that she drank coffee all day, and she was drinking more sucrose than she realized.

Consider these facts about sugar:

- It's a powerful trigger food for many and also a common Formula Buster.

- It's in many foods, even those savory non-dessert ones. Because people don't know this, they may consume more than they realize. These obstacles will seriously hinder your success.

FORMULA FACTOR: HOW MUCH SUGAR?

Here's an effective way to visualize how much sugar Brenda was consuming.

You know what a sugar cube looks like—exactly four grams of sugar. If Brenda read labels consistently, she would notice the sugar grams and divide those by four. She would be shocked to find the total number of sugar cubes in one cup of her creamer-filled coffee.

The flavored, sweetened, liquid creamer has five grams of sugar in a tablespoon. There are four tablespoons in a quarter cup. Four tablespoons x 5 grams of sugar = 20 grams of sugar! Brenda was consuming 20 grams of sugar in each cup of coffee. When Brenda drank five cups of coffee each day, she actually consumed one hundred grams of sugar:

$$\frac{\textbf{100 Sugar Grams}}{\textbf{4 grams per sugar cube}} = \textbf{25 Sugar Cubes}$$

If she took those sugar cubes and stacked them up in a pretty design, she could see how much sugar she consumed each day in her coffee.

Are you surprised? Brenda was, too.

Remember, you can do this exercise with any food. All you need is the nutrition label, which will show the grams of sugar.

FORMULA BUSTER #11: LIVING TO EAT

"Action expresses priorities." —Mahatma Gandhi

It's good to emphasize special eating occasions and prepare for them with all your heart. This is one of life's pleasures. My point is to maintain a sense of priority about your eating so food doesn't dominate your life.

Once a healthy diet is routine for you, you won't have to pay much attention to it because it's already a habit. When you've reached this place, then you have become emotionally detached from the need to have that constant overemphasis on the food. You are eating to live.

MELISSA'S STORY

Melissa was overweight and had few friends. She really didn't care about companionship. All she wanted to do was come home from work every day, be alone, and eat. She was very particular about her food and used this as an excuse to avoid socializing.

Vegetables had to be cooked a specific way, meat had to be spiced just right, pasta had to be cooked to the perfect tenderness, cereal must be served with whole milk, and coffee was not palatable without generous additions of half-and-half. She also loved butter, bacon bits, shredded cheese, and croutons. Finally, dessert always had to follow, especially at night. Every meal was an event.

Needless to say, when Melissa decided to lose weight, she had a hard time changing. She felt severely deprived if she couldn't have all the foods she felt she needed to be happy. She was depressed at the thought of giving up so much.

Food was everything to her. She lived to eat.

FORMULA FACTOR: EATING TO LIVE

Melissa came to realize her meals needed to become as routine as brushing her teeth, with the focus on health and the details forgotten.

While she continued to celebrate special occasions with excellent meals, she began to maintain a sense of priority about her eating. Food no longer dominated her life.

She learned the basics of nutrition and made meals simpler and more routine. She no longer had to pay much attention to food preparation once she made healthy eating a habit.

It was not easy, but in time, Melissa became emotionally detached from her constant overemphasis on food. She now ate to live.

Change is hard. It's easy to resist it. Melissa needed a friend or social group of people who shared the desire to lose weight so they could exchange support and provide mutual accountability.

As Melissa moved toward a better eating plan, she realized how much time she wasted focusing on food. All of a sudden, she had time on her hands.

If you found yourself in this place, what could you do? Here are a few ideas:

- Join a gym to go to classes and get to know the participants.
- Select a volunteer endeavor. Choose a regular time to engage, where you see the same people.
- Read classical literature each day to enrich your mind. You can buy used books for almost nothing online.
- Schedule a chat session with a friend at the same time each week.

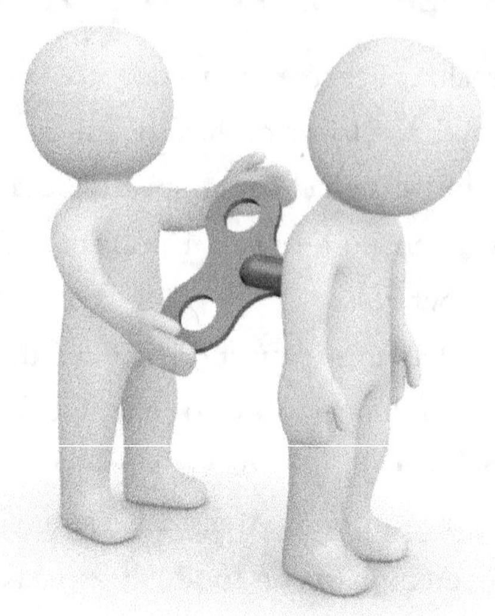

FORMULA BUSTER #12: WANING MOTIVATION

"People often say that motivation doesn't last. Well, neither does bathing—that's why we recommend it daily." —Zig Ziglar

Weight loss takes time and dedication. Like a fire that needs continual refueling, your initial motivation will burn low if its flame is not rekindled from time to time.

Your motivation may be the single most important element in a successful weight-loss program. Whether your goal is to improve your health, your appearance, or your life in general, you had a specific reward in mind when you began. The spark might be an upcoming wedding or other special event, a doctor's diagnosis of pre-diabetes, or simply an unguarded glimpse in the mirror.

Our initial success often acts as its own incentive. Even a small achievement may fan the inner fire needed to continue making emotionally and physically healthy changes.

But after the first flush of victory, when our clothing becomes looser and we feel more energetic and alive, we may be tempted to relax our efforts. How do we recapture the energy to press on? This may be the ultimate hurdle to overcome.

We've all experienced times when we forced ourselves to start a program and were unable to continue. Because we had no internal force to spur us on, we soon failed. Even as a fire cannot continue to burn without oxygen, we must find an internal source of energy and a higher purpose in order to stay motivated.

What does it take to stimulate you to stay on your program? There seems to be no cut-and-dried formula, even as there is none for your diet. Nothing is more frustrating than knowing you need to lose weight and finding yourself unwilling to make the necessary lifestyle changes. I see motivation as a beautiful and mysterious lover I must court all the days of my life. When I think it's mine, it slips away, and I fall into the dust of humility and self-rejection—an all-too-familiar pattern.

Whatever your objective may be, you will have to find a way to self-motivate. What sparks your curiosity, what do you seek answers for, and what do you deeply desire? If you are motivated, you will persist until you get results, even though you may stumble.

Motivation gives us energy and a sense of purpose. It's a prize worth seeking in itself.

WHAT MOTIVATED ME TO LOSE WEIGHT?

"Motivation is a fire from within. If someone else tries to light that fire under you, chances are it will burn very briefly." —Stephen R. Covey

When I was in such emotional pain, I almost forgot about how unhappy I was with my body. I simply wanted relief from my distress. I was lonely, with no one to talk to about my problems. My eating was out of control. I hated my lack of self-discipline and willpower.

I ate everything I could get my hands on, always in secret. When I wasn't eating, my mind obsessed about food until I could blindly stuff my face once again. Eating was no longer an act of survival. It became a tool of destruction.

The longer I continued this path, the more self-loathing I had. I could see myself drowning, and I didn't want to die, but neither did I know how to save myself.

At this point, God intervened.

What led me to walk on the Seine River that day? How did I notice the American Church in Paris? What made me walk inside?

The surface of the large reception table in the lobby was covered with brochures, advertisements, postcards, business cards, and other items big and small. In all this assortment, how was I led to the inside of one newsletter, where the classified ads were? How did my eyes fall upon the advertisement for *Overeaters Anonymous*? I saw more than a name and contact phone number and knew the words were written for me, "Is the way you eat affecting the way you live?" I'll never forget them.

"Yes! Help me," my spirit proclaimed. I was hooked. Someone up there reached down from the heavens and stood me on my feet. I'll believe until the day I die that God sent me to that place.

Why am I talking about God leading me somewhere when this section is about motivation? Because this is where it all began for me. My energy to change had to come from a place of infinite love, of knowing I had a Keeper and sensing He had my back. I needed spiritual support, and this moment was the beginning of a lifetime of change.

Attendance at meetings was a start, but there was much more I needed to do:

- Acknowledge my helpless situation and inability to fix myself.
- Accept there was Someone outside of myself who could help me.
- Ask Him many times a day to do so.

- Learn to live a life of introspection.

- Accumulate tools to help me face perplexing situations, difficult people, and my imperfect past.

- Change my lifestyle in order to become free from unhealthy eating patterns and mental obsessions.

- Learn balanced nutrition and the size of regular portions.

- Establish and maintain a habit of consistent exercise.

FORMULA FACTOR: INTERNALLY GENERATED MOTIVATION

"Motivation is what gets you started. Habit is what keeps you going."
—Jim Rohn

These principles may sound daunting, but if you sincerely desire to change your life and diligently apply them, I believe you too will lose weight and keep it off. Even more, you will achieve emotional, physical, and spiritual health. This is less a matter of rigorous effort than of releasing unhealthy thoughts and habits. The prize of dreams fulfilled awaits you!

QUESTIONS

1. Do you hold in your feelings, rather than express them in healthy ways? If you stuff down your emotions with food, this is a method of control.

Challenge: Start by writing each day in the morning. Fill up one 8 ½" x 11" sheet of paper. Purge those feelings before you begin your day. Get in touch with you.

2. Are you socially isolated, instead of regularly connecting with others?

This is most likely from a fear of rejection. It may be easier to not even try, rather than face the possibility of someone not liking you. Don't let your past hurts control your present.

Challenge: Get involved with a social group that meets regularly, perhaps to play cards, learn about the Bible, or pursue something else that interests you.

3. Do you have a fear of emotional intimacy with others? This may stem from issues of feeling abandoned when you were a child.

Challenge: Small groups at church are great ways to open up in a safe environment. Sign up for one and attend weekly.

4. Do you lack introspection? Can you explore yourself more deeply to gain understanding and self-compassion? You may have a fear of emotional pain here, and this can paralyze you from healing.

Challenge: Use your journal to ask God to reveal these inner truths to you and to give you courage to face your feelings. You may need to see a professional counselor to help you walk through old traumas. You must feel your emotions in order to heal them.

5. Are you reluctant to face the pain of your past? Yes, everyone—including you—has regrets. This is similar to the previous question, but with more self-awareness. You may rationalize that self-examination is pointless, what's done is done and you can't do anything about it. Not so! In fact, it's possible that by not addressing certain issues, you are perpetuating unwanted behavior in your life.

Challenge: Pray for the boldness and willingness to begin. Take one action today toward forgiveness of others and of yourself, moving you closer to this goal.

6. When you are hurting, do you rely on overeating for comfort, instead of reaching out to a friend? You must change your unhealthy responses to break new ground in your life. This is the only way out of the dangerous trap of isolation.

Challenge: Try voice calling (not texting) someone next time you are tempted to binge.

7. Do you consider yourself different from others, and therefore justify eating more food than you need? This must be exposed as a lie. You need perspective. Chances are you have separated yourself from others, and you have more in common with them than you think.

Challenge: You might need more social interaction and less time alone for a few weeks, to be less tempted by the food. Fill up your schedule, especially for those times you typically succumb to overeating.

DRIVE REDUCTION THEORY[lix]

"Motivation is like food for the brain. You cannot get enough in one sitting. It needs continual and regular top-up's." —Peter Davies

While the drive-reduction theory of motivation was once a dominant force in psychology, it is largely ignored today. Despite this fact, I'm bringing it up to make you aware of something that may be controlling your unwanted behavior with food.

According to American psychologist Clark Hull, who developed and popularized this theory in 1943, humans have internal biological needs that motivate us to perform a certain way. A drive creates an unpleasant state that demands relief. These needs, or drives, were defined by Hull as internal states of arousal or tension that must be reduced.

A prime example would be the internal feeling of hunger, motivating us to eat. According to this theory, we are driven to reduce this tension so we may maintain a sense of internal calmness.

Let's examine this analysis:

You have emotional discomfort from something that happened recently or perhaps long ago. You feel a compulsion to eat in order to relieve the uncomfortable feeling. You may experience these feelings on a daily, near daily, or periodic basis. Regardless, they occur regularly enough to cause you problems with your weight.

Overeating may be the tool you use to create the comfort you so desperately seek. Unfortunately, it backfires for those of us who misuse or abuse the luxury. For normal folks, an occasional bout of gluttony does no harm. For me—and maybe you—it works against us. Here's the healthy sequence:

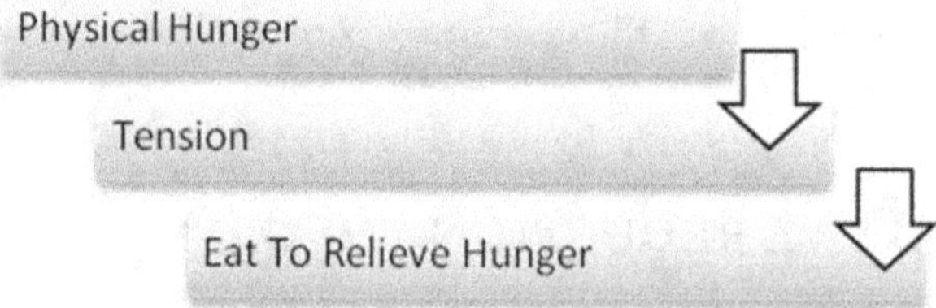

And the unhealthy one:

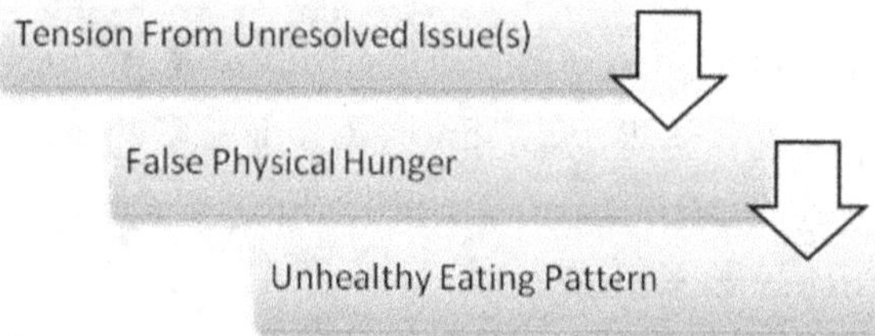

Can you see how your motive to eat can be controlled by emotional discomfort?

How did our lines get so crossed? At what point did we develop the method of eating as a way to experience relief from pain? When did the tension precede and even provoke the craving for food?

BELLE'S STORY

In the 1930's, many Americans were destitute. Belle was born in this Depression Era and developed a mindset of scarcity because there was little food and work.

Her brother was her mother's favorite. So not only was the family hungry and desperate for work to put food on the table, Belle was also emotionally starved for her mother's affection. This sting of rejection set the tone for her childhood, and food became her comfort.

Once an adult, Belle hopelessly accepted the belief she would be overweight the rest of her life. The weight began to take its toll when both knees needed replacement and back problems ensued. She was plagued with low energy and low self-esteem.

Her doctor confronted her with the results of her blood tests and implored her to change her lifestyle and eating habits. He warned she would soon need a wheelchair if she didn't take immediate action. This was her wake-up call.

One day, Belle was led to a church where she felt spiritually comfortable. She could grow in the Lord there. She met other women and felt validated and loved through these relationships. The healing from the pain of her past began, and she experienced forgiveness and compassion for her mother.

The hurts and bad habits Belle had developed through her life needed to be changed in order for her to lose weight. This was a two-part process:

Inside—emotional healing and working through her fears. She had to identify those things that compelled her to overeat, face them head-on, and courageously try new patterns of behavior.

Outside—education on nutritional balance and portion control, and learning new habits to create healthy meals and be physically active on a regular basis. She needed instruction from outside sources.

POSITIVE THINKING—THE PROVEN WAY TO ACHIEVE

How will you succeed when you don't really want to do the required work to realize that goal? For example, your goal may be to be thinner, but you may not necessarily want to exercise every day for fifteen minutes. However, you want to feel energized, so you do it anyway.

It is much easier to do anything when you clearly know the reasons why you're doing it.

HOMEWORK

The following three steps combine motivation and positive thinking. Personalize them in your notebook. Place them at your daily quiet time area. Read them each day *before* doing anything else. Don't allow yourself to get sidetracked.

1. **Decide what you want.** Many people cruise through life not even knowing what they want. They simply react to what comes along, either by accepting it or by rejecting it. They remain victims of circumstance and don't even know it. As such, they don't realize they have a choice. You do have the power to choose what you want. Take control over your mind and be specific.

2. **Why do you want it?** This is your carrot on the stick. Your reasons to have, be, or do something must be strong enough to carry you through the path to your goal. This list will keep you from giving up, because you know you will eventually achieve your dream.

3. **Use motivation and positive thinking together.** You can utilize visualization techniques, Bible verses, and positive affirmations to create the good feelings you will have when you achieve your goal.

THERE IS NO MAGIC ANSWER

I saw a friend recently I hadn't seen in over 6 months. He had lost a substantial amount of weight, so I couldn't resist asking him how much he lost and how he did it. He said he simply stopping eating bread, sugar, and junk food (a pretty good program by most standards).

I asked him what pushed him forward. He replied, "I don't know!"

I pressed him, "C'mon, you must have had *something* happen to persuade you!"

He explained, "I got sick of looking at myself and feeling the way I felt. Something clicked inside me, and I was ready to go."

His response was frustrating for me. I expected a magic solution or some consistent thread I could piece together like a jigsaw puzzle. He didn't give me the mystic answer, nor have I found one since. I'm afraid it will always be this way.

Some things in life are like that. You and I will have to reinvent the wheel for ourselves. We can gather information, wisdom, and experiences from others. We can share and commiserate with those we trust. But ultimately, through counsel with God, we have to go it alone.

What isn't known about motivation could fill volumes of books, but most everyone will agree on one thing: *it's as individual as you are.* Read on for some ideas you can apply today.

Motivation is as individual as you are.

SHORT-TERM AMBITION

Creating temporary drive isn't too hard. Consider New Year's resolutions. Remember how energized you were to succeed? What happened to those goals? Did you start out strong but fizzle out in a week or two?

If you can get your program off to a good start, here are some things you can try to get you through tough spots that are sure to come:

- Temporarily hire specialists. Select those who inspire you and have the credentials to help you get results. This outside help can drive you. However, few of us want to keep these appointments forever. You may not be able to afford specialists indefinitely. (If you are, lucky you!) Most clients prefer to train for a period of time and move on.

- Designate a date in the future—a vacation, wedding, graduation, or reunion—that will give you the enthusiasm needed to reach your goal.

- Sign up for a class in yoga, dance, aerobics, or another physical activity where you can meet others and generate *esprit de corps* (a feeling of pride, fellowship, and common loyalty shared by the members of a particular group).

LONG-TERM PERSISTENCE

If you stick with a weight-loss program long and consistently enough, you will see results. Sometimes this can be all the reason you need to reach your goal. However, what happens when you enter the maintenance phase? You need to find ways to keep those pounds from creeping back on.

Long-term impetus is difficult, because it must be internally generated and maintained. Since there is no formula for this, you must find your own.

Think for a moment about how the advertising industry markets a product. They know people buy products because of their *emotional appeal*—as if the item itself would satisfy some internal need. This is the realm where *your* fire needs to happen.

Goals to have good health, to be attractive, and to have self-confidence are all internally based. These come from positive feelings, which are the most effective and long-lasting catalysts.

By contrast, ambition can be generated through fear, which is negative. "My husband will leave me if I don't lose weight!" Unfortunately, this might work for a while, but probably won't have a long-term effect.

HOMEWORK

What excites you? If you don't know, you need to find out now! Get your notebook and answer the following:

- What is your biggest mental block or fear?

- What do you desire most in life?

- When do you have "get up and go?"

- Strong emotions of any type are good indicators of your passion. List one and trace it to a wish you have for yourself.

- Write down anything you believe would contribute to your self-actualization.

Here are some additional ways people have developed determination. Try these to see if they work for you:

- Reading fitness magazines to see beautiful bodies, get workout suggestions, and trending ideas related to the industry.

- Reading books to learn more about specific areas of nutrition, fitness, or how to generate internal drive.

- Attending performances that involve athletic prowess, including ballet, acrobatics, modern dance, sports, the Olympics, and fitness competitions.

- Participating in your gym's weight-loss or fitness contest.

- Taking a nutrition or personal training course. This might be a way to meet others interested in the same topic.

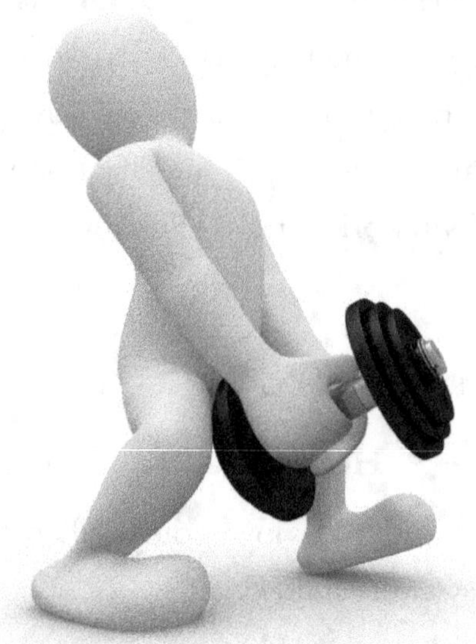

FORMULA BUSTER #13: RESISITANCE TO EXERCISE

"He has all the virtues I dislike and none of the vices I admire."
—Winston Churchill

Regular physical activity isn't an option, but a necessity! We all know the benefits of exercise. No matter where we go, we are bombarded with them, *ad nauseum*. The dangers of slothfulness are far worse. So to shake things up, following are seven *bummers* about being lazy:

- Makes maintaining weight loss more difficult
- Increases potential for health conditions and diseases
- Opens the door to depression[lx][lxi][lxii]
- Lowers energy
- Creates sleep problems
- Lowers libido

- Decreases quality of life

To avoid this bad health trap, you have several options:

OPTION 1: Do something to move your body every day.

This is for you couch potatoes, sedentary folk, or those of you who hate to sweat. Physical movement feels good and is positive. Your body and mind need it.

Physical exertion combats depression. It's uplifting due to your increase in metabolism and will help you reach your weight loss goals sooner. The best part? It keeps your body young!

I'm not suggesting you purchase a gym membership, buy home equipment, or join a running club. I am asking you to change your viewpoint about moving your body. Look for ways to fit physical activity into your current lifestyle.

Some examples might be:

- Gardening or other creative yard work
- Nature walk or walk your dog (they need exercise too)
- Mall walk and window-shop with a friend
- A leisurely bike ride
- Dance to music as you sweep your deck or patio outside
- Swim and splash in a pool with a child

The list could go on and on. Make the activity fun. You don't need to spend extra money or time to make physical activity part of your current lifestyle.

OPTION 2: For die-hard fitness enthusiasts.

If you love working out, you are already doing regular exercise. However, even as a diet needs to be nutritionally balanced, so does a fitness program.

Too much high-intensity *anything* is not an ideal fitness program. Your body gets tired and needs a break. Offset intense days with periods of rest or flexibility training. On the other hand, a straight diet of yoga isn't ideal either, because the heart isn't getting enough stress to be conditioned.

If you do only weight training, your muscles will become shorter and less flexible, and your heart won't get enough conditioning. Doing only cardio with no weight or flexibility training can result in a flabby, shapeless body. Seems like we can't win for losing, right? No!

Regardless what option you choose, your body craves balance in all things. When you combine the right amounts of effort from the following list, you will look and feel your best:

- Cardiovascular workouts
- Strength training
- Flexibility and stretching
- Balance, stability, and range-of-motion activities

Let's look at some ways you might go about this. Keep in mind these are only examples and not specific suggestions or recommendations.

FORMULA FACTOR: COMMIT TO STAYING ACTIVE

LORENA'S STORY

Lorena is a fifty-two-year-old woman, married with a ten-year-old child. She has been active for years and always enjoyed great health and vitality. But her child's increased activities take most of her time every day and evening. Recently, she began menopause, and her energy sagged. This created a dilemma for her, knowing she wanted to maintain all these activities. Her key was determination and insistence to have what she desired. Here's what she did.

Her fatigue needed to be addressed first. She talked with friends in her age group and heard about hormone replacement therapy. Curious, she began reading up on the various types and decided on the direction she wanted to take.

Finding the right doctor took some experimentation. Lorena needed to feel comfortable sharing her physical needs, as well as trusting this professional's judgment about her health.

It took a couple of years and great expense. At first, she inquired at her general practitioner's to receive blood work. Her doctor told her everything was normal. She knew otherwise. She tried again the following year with the same result.

Frustrated, Lorena shared her experience with her OB-GYN. He ordered more blood work. Not surprisingly, her numbers came back low, and she was given hormone replacement therapy. She asked why she was unable to get her normal doctor to do anything. He responded that, "GPs don't do hormones." In any case, she found a method she was happy with and stuck with it.

Now that the energy issue was somewhat resolved, she focused on prioritizing her activity. A friend meets her three times a week to do strength training and yoga in the morning.

This works great when her daughter is at school. However, she needs more—at least five days of movement per week is preferable for post-menopausal women if they want to stay at a healthy weight. Also, her friend sometimes cancels. She needs an alternate plan for those days too.

She decides to do cardio alone on other days. If her friend cancels, Lorena will get an additional day of heart conditioning in lieu of the workouts with her friend. It's all good!

By making daily exercise a priority, Lorena has worked these into her regular lifestyle:

- Cardiovascular—the days she doesn't meet with her friend

- Strength training—meeting with her fitness buddy
- Yoga for flexibility, stretching, balance, stability, and range of motion

RACHEL'S STORY

Rachel is an eighty-year-old woman, widowed, living with a sedentary roommate. She's a writer and works at her desk. She develops tight chest and shoulder muscles. In fact, she gets stiff all over from sitting for hours at a time. Combined with her age, she should emphasize strength training (for joints) and flexibility (for tightness) in her fitness program.

Lucky for her, she has a little dog, a built-in incentive to get out and walk. Certainly, he needs to get out each day, and Rachel will be doing herself some good at the same time. Walking lubricates the joints of the lower body, increases circulation for the heart, and is a fantastic precursor to a flexibility session.

How else can she add the other elements for a great fitness program? Being an innovative and resourceful person, she has arranged to work with a personal trainer in exchange for some editing.

Challenges remain, however. She only has one session a week with the trainer. This trade is only temporary. Once the arrangement ends, Rachel will need to take this knowledge and apply it herself.

Also, as a retired person on a fixed income, spending money to stay fit is not a good option.

Above all, once a week isn't enough for Rachel's muscles to stay supple. Although she's still searching for ways to fill this gap, here are some ideas she could try:

- Seek out a massage therapist or trainer for another trade
- Search You-Tube for videos on senior fitness
- Purchase DVD's online for "no-equipment" home workouts
- Find a neighbor with a dog and walk together at the same time each morning

- Find a no-cost church group that meets weekly to do a variety of fun and engaging body mechanics

Rachel's greatest asset is, as a retiree, she can make her own schedule. She can work out any time during the day or evening she chooses. She has some physical limitations, but she's learning how to overcome them with the trainer's help.

Despite her age, Rachel has achieved remarkable success in making these activities part of her regular lifestyle:

- Cardiovascular—most days, walking her dog
- Strength, flexibility, and range of motion—with her trainer

EMMA'S STORY

Emma is a forty-four-year-old woman with a full-time job. She is married to a sedentary, smoking, exercise-averse husband. They have no children.

I love this example, because Emma has so many obstacles to her fitness. You may think I'm crazy for saying so, but I actually like finding solutions to problems—especially other people's!

In addition to the issues mentioned, Emma had back surgery a few years ago wherein several vertebrae were fused. She also has power of attorney for her elderly mother, who lives in assisted living nearby. Her mom needs help from time to time, and this obligation frequently interferes with Emma's daily fitness routine.

Lazy Hubby's lifestyle is so different from Emma's. He doesn't seem to mind not taking care of his body and health. Unfortunately, their blended lifestyles have taken a toll on her, and she is plump. Since she has lived like this for many years, she does what she can and accepts the bad with the good.

Time is undoubtedly the biggest challenge for Emma, with her demanding job and the unpredictable needs of an elderly mother. How does she manage to exercise?

During the week, Emma shuts her office down at lunch, kicks her pumps off, and puts on sneakers. She hangs her jacket behind her door and treks at a fast clip to the company fitness center on the other side of the building. Once there, she does a variety of strength training at the gym's circuit. Yes, she gets sweaty most days, but she has learned to accept it. She keeps extra clothes, hairspray, and other essentials in her office for those days when she needs them.

To address her back limitation, she trained with a certified personal trainer until she knew how to use weights safely and effectively without compromising her bone health.

Emma's daily plan has another benefit—stress reduction and a break from the office monotony. She always returns refreshed.

In the evening, she attends to her husband's and mother's needs. Emma enjoys a large house and has a dedicated exercise room. It contains a treadmill, some weights, mats, and a large screen monitor with a DVD player. Emma has a library of yoga DVDs and squeezes this training in on most weekends.

Fortunately, her husband doesn't demand gourmet meals during the week, and they eat leftovers or at restaurants. But during the weekend, they let their culinary juices flow. They have late night guests over for multiple-course dinners. Desserts always follow. Being avid foodies, this is their lifestyle.

Although Emma does well during the week, she does much damage over the weekends. As she ages and her metabolism slows more each year, her weight creeps up.

Her resourcefulness has helped her overcome her sedentary lifestyle and the demands of her job and family:

- Cardiovascular—her walks to the gym
- Strength training—the circuits during the week
- All others—yoga DVDs during the weekend

SUMMARY

All this may sound overwhelming. True, it may be at first, but once you know and embrace these basics, you'll be on your way to a healthy body for the rest of your life. The confusing part is there is so much to choose from, and that's a good thing.

You are reading this book to develop your own formula for long-term weight loss. This is simply part of that same formula. With a little effort, you can find a great fitness plan that works for you and fits into your lifestyle.

Be aware, however, that if something works for you today, it might not fit tomorrow. Limitations due to age, medical issues, moving to another town, getting another job, having a child, and many other life-changing events will affect how and what you do for physical activity. Again, as I counseled you about your diet, be open-minded about periodically altering your exercise program.

FORMULA BUSTER #14: INCONSISTENCY

"Good ideas are common—what's uncommon are people who will work hard enough to bring them about." —Ashleigh Brilliant

One of the most important gifts we can give ourselves regarding our eating habits is consistency. This can be a challenge at times, but if we stay positive, we shouldn't have too much of a problem maintaining our formula while juggling special events.

Many people are able to reach their desired weight by following the 80/20 rule. With this plan, you adhere to your formula eighty percent of the time and give yourself freedom the remaining twenty percent.

SARAH'S STORY

Sarah has succeeded well with her program. Most weeks, she works all or most of the principles in this book about eighty percent of the time and eats a clean, healthy diet Sunday through Thursday.

However, one weekend, she splurged a little too much on sugar. On Friday night, she went on a date and ordered a large serving of ice cream. The following evening, approximately twenty-four hours later, she craved sugar once again, so she gave in and bought a piece of cake at the grocery store. On Sunday night, at the exact same time, she found herself obsessed with the desire for sweets.

Suddenly, she checked herself, aware she was backsliding on her program.

Her original plan was to give herself freedom with the sugars on Friday and Saturday. On Sundays, she'd resume her healthy eating.

Normally, she is more careful about what sweets she consumes on her "cheat days." Also, she usually eats them after her meal, when her body is already processing proteins, fats, and carbohydrates. Any sugar eaten is offset by these other nutrients, and the effect on her body is not as strong as if she were to eat dessert on an empty stomach. This is an important point to remember, since physiology plays such a large part in your cravings.

The stronger the urge, the weaker you become, and the more likely you will be to eat something you know you shouldn't have. If you know your triggers, you will be able to protect yourself most of the time. You won't always be able to avoid slip-ups, but your chances of long-term success will be much better.

Sarah realized she was in danger of regaining all the weight she'd lost. Her body screamed for more sugar. Her choices were either to give in to the craving once more, perpetuating the cycle for another twenty-four hours, or to abstain and be uncomfortable while she suffered withdrawal. At this point, the craving was even stronger because the sugar she ate over the last two days was so powerful. It might not have been so bad if her desserts were sugar-free frozen yogurt with nuts on top, a muffin with a glass of skim milk, or a tall, non-fat latte with biscotti.

She knew the sugar cravings would return on a daily basis until she buckled under and went "cold turkey." She also knew saying, "No" would take effort.

She recognized the insanity of playing "Sugar Russian Roulette" and forced herself to endure the necessary physical discomfort. She succeeded in dealing with this situation, and she is able to preserve the eighty percent healthy eating pattern, as well as her long-term weight loss.

Can you do what she did? Can you identify the foods that trigger such cravings? What would you do in her situation?

FORMULA FACTOR: CONSISTENCY

In order for you to be successful at losing and maintaining your goal weight, you will have to abstain from certain foods temporarily—or even indefinitely. Your priority is to stick to your formula, and your job is to know which foods you can safely eat and which you cannot.

Take out insurance to protect yourself. Allow a treat from time to time, but be *selective* about what and when you eat it.

COMPENSATION AS PUNISHMENT

In order to maintain your weight or at least not *gain* weight, you will need to plan your food vacations and compensate for them somehow. The more planning we do in advance, the more likely we will be to maintain our weight.

What are your plans for the weekend? Are you going to a party or to a fancy restaurant? What about the upcoming holidays? The family celebration later this year? How will you eat in those situations? Do you have a plan?

It's all too easy not to face this problem, and to not bother yourself with a plan. "I have too many other things to do," you think. "I'll worry about the consequences tomorrow."

When reality hits and the scales begin moving upward, you may try to make up for your diet deviations by limiting yourself. That doesn't sound so bad in itself, but over time, this will result in yo-yo dieting. Not such a good plan!

Compensation as punishment can take many forms. Here are a few harmful ways people punish themselves after they have over-indulged:

- Crash dieting
- Over-exercising
- Swearing off certain foods

These tactics might be temporarily effective in undoing some mistakes made with food. The problem is few lifestyle changes have really been made. The behaviors that put the weight on our bodies are still there. This is a negative way of dealing with the situation.

Read on, for a *healthier alternative*.

Consider your schedule again. A good way to prepare for these events is to plan for them in advance. If you do this, you will increase your self-discipline and motivation.

Always set consistent boundaries for yourself, such as eating before you go out in order to strengthen your willpower. Otherwise, you may consider these "food vacations." Three or four in one week will quickly sabotage your program.

JESSE'S STORY

Jesse is planning to attend a company dinner at a resort one weekend and knows he will drink cocktails, eat a four-course dinner, and enjoy a dessert buffet. This is a fun event, and he looks forward to a food vacation.

If he plans ahead, he might eat fewer carbohydrates and fats during the day of the event. He could even do this for two days before the event, if he felt it would help maintain his weight.

In this way, he is adjusting his lifestyle prior to receiving the reward. This is the most motivating and energizing way toward success. He has already done the work beforehand.

If you learn to balance your food intake and output, you will never have a weight problem again.

The self-discipline to prepare for your food vacation should be taken in advance. It makes no sense to pay the price after you have received the reward for anything, since that is demotivating and discouraging.

PHILLIP'S STORY

Phillip is planning a weeklong vacation. He can compensate by moderately dieting and increasing his exercise frequency a week or two before leaving town.

Another way he can attain balance is by being more active on vacation. Walking tours, an elaborate fitness room, and body surfing are all fun experiences and will keep him in great shape. These trips are the best ones, because they combine recreation with fitness.

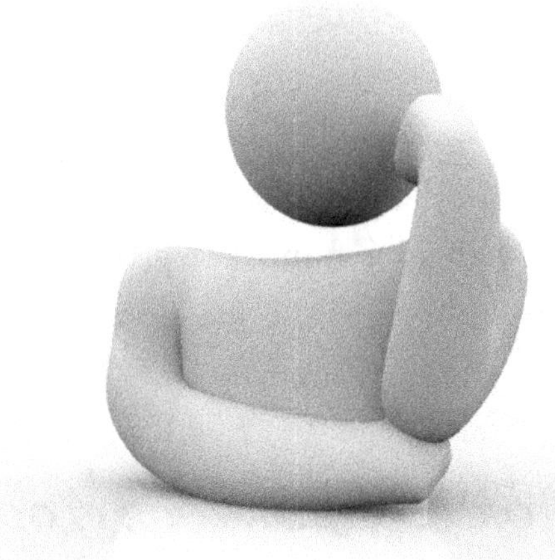

FORMULA BUSTER #15: CALORIE CONFUSION

"If confusion is the first step to knowledge, I must be a genius."
—Larry Leissner

Have you ever felt frustrated about all the conflicting nutritional information you read? One day, a certain food is "good" and another "bad." Almost the next day, the foods proclaimed bad are now okay. One article says one thing, then another written on practically the same day says the opposite. All this conflicting information can confuse people, and many have abandoned any attempt at dieting.

What is all this? How are we supposed to help ourselves with this mess of data?

As an example, we know that all foods have calories. Some dieters believe they only need to count the total number they consume each day, and what they eat is not so important.

Others subscribe to the theory that caloric values do not matter. Instead, they allow themselves the freedom to eat, but only certain types of food. Or, they may eat freely of some foods and eliminate others entirely for the limited duration of their diet.

The truth is neither belief is accurate. Both will affect your weight-loss goals and need to be considered.

I hope this section will help give you the information you need to make definite headway with your formula. I promise to refrain from as much jargon as I can and only focus on the direct impact on your body, without confusing you with too much detail.

FORMULA FACTOR: CONTROL YOUR BLOOD SUGAR [lxiii]

I may be oversimplifying things by saying if you can control your blood sugar levels, you can lose weight. There are many ways to approach a diet, but if I were to give you one lesson, this would be it.

Once I understood how balancing my blood sugar worked, I was able to make wise choices and avoid poor ones. I began eating foods that would encourage this balance. I started to understand the importance of moderate portions. I also monitored when and what I ate. This has enabled me to maintain my weight for over thirty years.

We have two important hormones that are key players in blood sugar control—insulin and glucagon. Both work together to maintain a steady glucose balance in your body. Too much of one or the other, or too little of either, wreak havoc on your energy and sense of well-being. They can cause you to gain or lose weight, depending on how you manipulate your diet.

INSULIN

When you eat, your body produces insulin to lower blood sugar. The energy you have will come from the food you just ate. Any excess calories you do not use will be stored in the liver, muscles, or fat cells. This is why you gain weight when you constantly overeat. Your body's natural balancing system is at work.

GLUCAGON

This hormone is a major participant, in that it moves energy out of fat cells for your daily use. Between meals, your body produces glucagon to keep your blood sugar steady. The energy you have will come from your liver, muscles, and fat cells. If you eat small, frequent, nutrient-dense meals—and don't overeat—you will lose weight over time.

INSULIN	GLUCAGON
Energy comes from blood stream	Energy comes from liver, muscles and fat cells (storage)
Stores excess and unused energy calories	Uses calories in storage for energy
Suppresses Glucagon	Suppresses Insulin

Have you ever eaten a dessert, sleeve of cookies, or box of crackers—only to crash at some point, and later crave the same thing again? This is because your body produced insulin to move those excess calories into your fat cells. When this happened, your blood sugar spiked (from all the consumed carbs) and then fell (once the insulin did its work). That's the crash you felt. This is the cycle you don't want, the one that will perpetuate cravings for junk and cause weight gain.

Certain foods, like the ones mentioned above, will create a surge in insulin. Also, any large, high-calorie meal, even if it is totally nutritious, can cause a spike.

In light of this information, this is how to experience continuing success with weight loss:

- Many small meals throughout the day
- Avoid processed carbohydrates (The next section will discuss in greater detail how to rank carbohydrates as they relate to blood sugar.)

Energy will come from both sources—the calories you eat and from your fat cells. Your metabolism will be evenly regulated, and you will feel great. You will also be happy because you're dropping unwanted pounds!

Chances are glucagon is a major participant in removing energy out of those fat cells for your daily use.

You might have the impression it would benefit you to encourage your body to produce glucagon only, with no insulin. Don't do it. You wouldn't feel well if you did, and that's putting it mildly.

Please don't adhere to an either-or mentality with these hormones. You need both to be healthy and feel good. They complement each other and work together synergistically for your optimal health.

UNDERSTANDING THE GLYCEMIC INDEX[lxiv]

Now that you have this information on insulin and glucagon, how can you apply it?

Many people believe that all carbohydrates end up as glucose in your body and claim that a calorie is a calorie—the source makes no difference. What a dieter needs to watch for, they say, are the total calories consumed in a day.

Others believe that all carbohydrates are bad for us—fattening, unhealthy, or evil obstacles to our success. Under this assumption, many dieters want to avoid them all.

The carbohydrates that actually *are* bad are the simplest ones (candy, desserts, alcohol). The ones that are good and should be eaten are the fibrous and starchy ones (fruits, vegetables, legumes, and whole grains).

Finally, others may think all carbs are equal, because bread, pasta, rice, and cereal are all pretty much alike. But the truth is not all carbs are created equally. Our bodies process different ones in a variety of ways.

While I don't want to bore you with too many facts, it's important to learn how various carbohydrates are metabolized by our bodies. This knowledge will help you make healthier choices and lead to success in weight loss and weight maintenance for life.

THE GLYCEMIC INDEX AS A TOOL

The glycemic index (GI) was originally created for diabetics as a way to determine which foods would be best for them. It has become popular because it's easy to understand. This simple measurement shows where carbohydrates fall in comparison with others (on a scale of 1-100), as well as their impact on our bodies.

A carbohydrate with a high glycemic index breaks down quickly during digestion and releases energy into the bloodstream rapidly. By contrast, a low one breaks down more slowly. This causes a gradual release of glucose, thus choosing carbohydrates with a lower GI helps maintain steady blood glucose levels throughout the day.

Choosing carbs with a lower GI helps maintain steady blood glucose levels.

Be aware, however, of the tool's limitations:

First, it doesn't take normal serving sizes into account. This means that 50 grams of a food might have a different effect on blood sugar than 100 grams of that same food.

Also, the GI is based on foods as if they were eaten in isolation. This is unrealistic, as most meals are a combination of several items.

This information will only give an idea of carbohydrates in relation to one another and will enable us to make the best food choices.

All this deeper nutritional knowledge will gradually give multiple benefits:

- Controlling hunger
- Maintaining energy levels
- Improving the way our bodies look
- Preventing a variety of health issues associated with frequent

and sustained spikes in blood sugar levels (like Type II diabetes and heart disease).

So if we choose our carbohydrates mostly from the low GI category, these foods will help us to not only lose excess weight, but they will also help maintain healthy blood sugar levels.

Examples of foods with a low GI (55 or less) include legumes, chickpeas, seeds, most intact whole grains (as contrasted with flour), most vegetables, fruits, and fructose.

Foods with a medium GI (56-69) include products containing whole-wheat flour or enriched wheat flour, pita bread, basmati rice, unpeeled boiled potatoes, grape juice, raisins, prunes, pumpernickel bread, regular ice cream, sucrose, and bananas.

Foods with a high GI (70-100) include white bread, most white rice, corn flakes, processed breakfast cereals, glucose, maltose, pretzels, and bagels.

Below is a sample of some common foods and their GIs.[lxv]

FOOD TYPE BY CATEGORY	GLYCEMIC INDEX (GLUCOSE = 100)	SERVING SIZE IN GRAMS
Bagel, white, frozen	72	70
Pita bread, whole wheat	57	1 Pocket
Cranberry Juice Cocktail	68	250
Orange juice	50	250
Cornflakes	81	30
Oatmeal	58	250
Whole wheat kernels	41	50
Skim milk	32	250
Nonfat yogurt, plain, artificial sweetener	14	220
Apple, average	38	120
Dates, dried	103	60
Peanuts	14	50
Spaghetti, white, boiled 20m	61	180
Lean Cuisine © French style chicken	36	

Microwave popcorn	72	20
Broccoli, cauliflower, celery	10-25	
Baked russet potato	85	150
Yam	37	150
Pizza, plain baked dough w/parmesan cheese and tomato sauce	80	100

LEGEND[lxvi]	
Hi GI	70 and above
Medium GI	56-69
Low GI	55 and below

Here's a link to look at another Glycemic Index chart:

http://www.nasm.org/trainer-resources/glycemic-index.

It may not have all foods on this list, but you can find other charts online. If you are looking for the GI on a specific food, you can search, "glycemic index for ___________."

FORMULA BUSTER #16: OUR HUMAN CONDITION

"When life gives you lemons, make orange juice and leave the world wondering how you did it." —Ritesh Sharma

I had always been a shy kid, but after my weight loss, I was more so than ever. Food, my coping tool, wasn't there to help me navigate life. I felt naked, exposed, and afraid. Being attractive was a scary experience. Men noticed me, and that frightened me. I also felt women acted hostile toward me for no reason. Were they mad because I was thin? Or was it something else? Maybe I was being paranoid.

I assumed confidence and social mobility would naturally follow my goal weight, but that didn't happen. It was soon clear I would have to reach out, take risks, and be uncomfortable at times, if I were to meet others and gain new friends.

I felt self-conscious and judged by others. In retrospect, I think I was judging myself. Even though I looked fine in a bathing suit, I felt even more uncomfortable going to a public pool. No way would I try sports or physical activities.

Gaining confidence has been a huge process for me. It is still a challenge at times.

Everyone has emotional problems that can make them feel distanced from others. This is a common human condition. For me, it was my eating problem.

FORMULA FACTOR: SELF-ACCEPTANCE

The important thing is what you do with the bad things that happen to you. You can hang on to these experiences and allow them to hold you back in life, or you can grow from them, help others, and have fun doing so.

The revelation that others have their own internal issues makes me feel more equal instead of feeling so inferior. We are all imperfect. Let's remember this so we can develop a love for humanity.

A mark of maturity is to realize this truth, accept yourself, and embrace your fellow humans despite their imperfections. Friendship is a gift when you can have a relationship knowing full well what the other's faults are. You can put their flaws aside and simply enjoy one another's company.

Contrast this with your relationship with God. Except He is perfect and He loves you unconditionally.

He accepts you just as you are, with all your imperfections. He does because He made you that way for a reason. It's your job to find out what He has planned for you in this world. That truth will unfold throughout your life, in your all-important quiet time each day.

FORMULA BUSTER #17: DISCONTENTMENT

"When it comes to life the critical thing is whether you take things for granted or take them with gratitude." —Gilbert K. Chesterton

When I started writing about Formula Busters, I knew I should include a chapter on gratitude vs. discontent. I would be negligent if I didn't write about this all-important topic.

Perhaps because I have struggled with an ungrateful mindset for much of my life, this needs to be a part of my book.

I didn't know much about the subject when I wrote my rough draft. I wrote a few paragraphs and considered them complete. However, when I began the lengthy editing process, I had to admit those few sentences were sorely inadequate.

Then I began to study the subject of contentment as a virtue. I found so much information I was ashamed I had not given it more attention. In fact, there is so much to write about on this topic, it is worthy of a book of its own.

I began to wonder if I should start the entire book with this as Chapter One or perhaps the Introduction. As I recognized contentment's value, I awakened to a new world with great potential...that begins with my outlook.

FORMULA FACTOR: CONTENTMENT AS A VIRTUE[lxvii]

The most important lesson to glean about contentment is that it's something you can learn and practice—just like your faith. It's not a thing you are given, or something that necessarily comes naturally. Although you work for it, it is ultimately a gift from God.

Contentment is something you can learn and practice.

Seek wisdom and study what it means to be content. This too, is a process. Be happy with your body today, rather than the results you want, for this is also a form of gratitude. Think of how far you have travelled, even if you've only begun your journey. You've made real progress!

Make a point not to grumble or complain about anything to anybody. What can you substitute for these thoughts when they come into your mind?

- Orally speak a Bible verse that counters the negative thought. Your subconscious mind will hear and eventually obey and believe.

- Get busy with something you need to do that day, or create something with your hands. Producing something of value is a positive action that will drown out any negativity.

- Avoid speaking dark thoughts about anything, even minor physical pains. These words create a negative atmosphere.

- Encourage others to talk about themselves, and listen to what they say.

Envy of others creates a spirit of discontent within you. Are you reading unwholesome magazines or books that stir the wrong desires? Are you watching TV programs or listening to music that makes you crave something you don't have?

You must look at all these things and be honest about the impact they have on your mind. Rid yourself of them, or at least limit them. You can wean yourself away from bad influences. Over time, you will be a happier, more contented person for doing so.

A craving for excess food is one way discontentment manifests itself in our lives. It shows we are not satisfied with the amount our bodies require. We want more than we need. This indicates we are seeking to fulfill ourselves in ways that are outside the will of God.

God doesn't want us to destroy ourselves. When we overeat for years, becoming obese and carrying unhealthy, excess weight, is this not self-destruction?

Contentment is a form of humility. It confesses God knows the better path for me than I do for myself. It also trusts Him to provide for my every need, so I need not be fearful of the future.

Cultivating a grateful heart is the best way to free yourself of discontentedness, restlessness, and dissatisfaction.

In contrast, thinking about what you don't have keeps you in a place of scarcity. Focusing on your fears can actually make them reality. If you dwell on negativity, you invite exactly those results.

How can you change your way of thinking?

- Ask God to transform your mind.[lxviii]

- Identify your deepest desires and work toward these goals each and every day.

- Make the decision to focus on what you truly want. Ignore all else. This is a huge step toward living right.

- Be grateful for what you have.

- Focus your energy on those things you control—your thoughts, health, possessions, etc. This will empower you to be successful in all areas of life.

Your weight loss and maintenance will be a by-product of changing from a lack of gratitude to a grateful heart.

Another excellent suggestion is to begin each day doing two things, regardless of how we feel:

- List twenty things you are grateful for.

- List five things you need to do that day. Starting with the one you want to do the least, complete them all.

These two things will turn your mind toward the positive. The first enables you to keep your eyes on what you have, rather than what you don't have. The second is the action part, actually doing something positive.

Both these exercises work in conjunction with each other to produce a grateful heart. I promise you will increase your energy and motivation to be even more productive than your list of five things. You'll accomplish more than you thought possible when you start your days this way!

You may not be at your goal weight, have the body you want, the material satisfaction, or the relationships you crave—yet—but you can be content with where you are today and be grateful.

You can appreciate the changes God is making in you—a willingness to stick with your formula, an open mind for new ideas, and the humility to take instruction from others.

Many have never taken these first steps to improve their lives. Unfortunately, they stay stuck indefinitely, perhaps until death. You are not one of them!

Even though some days may be hard, also know the good days are still ahead. As long as you keep moving forward with a good attitude, you will succeed. You will win!

FORMULA BUSTER #18: ALL-OR-NOTHING MENTALITY

"Complete abstinence is easier than perfect moderation." —St. Augustine

Do you believe a diet must be strict to be effective? No cheating whatsoever, no desserts, no treats, no restaurants, and no ________________________ (you fill in the blank)?

For example, if you usually drink a glass of wine every night, with this all-or-nothing mentality, you might believe you must now abstain completely. If your favorite snack is chips and salsa, you may think they're taboo, at least until after you've lost weight. If you love to celebrate birthdays, you may think you cannot enjoy a piece of cake anymore.

You can live without alcohol. You can't live without food. Not drinking is an option for anyone. Not eating isn't. Because of this hard fact, we have to look more closely at the reasons behind the eating, both in a physical and an emotional sense. The awareness we have will guide us to our best choices.

The issue shouldn't be whether you limit yourself or not. The real question is, "What will happen to me when I do eat this? Will I lose control after I eat/drink one serving?" Or perhaps, "I may have control for a while after eating this, but in time, my defenses will falter."

You see, it's not *what* you eat that's the problem, but rather what it *does* to you. You must observe your past behavior and make some hard decisions rooted in honesty. Chances are there may be some things you shouldn't eat at all.

Ever.

Or at least, for the time being.

Remember my story about Francoise and the bread? Really, I thought I could not survive without it! Well, that was thirty-three years ago, and I still stay away from the stuff. I know how I tend to get when I eat it, and my behavior hasn't changed in all this time.

Every now and then I do a little experimentation, but the result is always the same: I tend to lose control, even after eating a few bites. My obsession with bread's delightful taste, texture, and fragrance returns. Every day I find myself craving some, and I feel depressed when I deny myself. If this reality doesn't keep me on the right path, nothing will.

Bread is one item for me that is "all or nothing"—or at least eaten *very* rarely. But I can occasionally indulge in other items without losing control, so there is a safe middle ground between the two extremes. It depends on your chemistry.

FORMULA FACTOR: MODERATION MENTALITY

This less-strict program accomplishes two things:

- You will lose weight, even if it is more slowly, than by a severely strict diet.
- You will change your lifestyle and be able to maintain the weight loss for life.

If you are trying to lose weight and want to enjoy a glass of wine each evening, why not try cutting it down to the weekends only, to Friday, Saturday, and Sunday? Are you able to stay consistent with this new schedule, not only to lose weight, but also to maintain it for the rest of your life? Or would you regard this experiment as a temporary one, looking forward to a time when you can drink without limitation? Only you can answer.

If you love to eat chips and salsa, can you skip a day and eat them every other day to begin your program? Then can you progress to once a week and be satisfied? If not, this particular food might be taking a more important role in your life than is healthy.

If you love birthday festivities, can you eat one moderately-sized piece of cake and be done with it? Or would you take home the leftovers and finish them off later that day?

If you enjoy baking, how easy is it to make something without eating batter or licking the bowl? Is this more of a temptation than you can handle right now?

Note I said, "Right now." I did not say, "Forever." How differently would you behave if you were to resist only this once, rather than think you had to abstain from something indefinitely?

This perspective on moderation can mean the difference between success and failure. Being too strict with anything is a recipe for disaster. Looking at something with a "forever" mentality sets you up for failure. Absolutes will get you nowhere but upset with yourself.

Being too strict with anything is a recipe for disaster.

Instead of completely abstaining from something you love, find a way to eat those things a little less frequently—if you honestly believe you can handle them.

This conversation may seem ambiguous, as if I'm advising strictness in one sentence and laxity in another. The truth is I *am* unclear, because there's one thing missing—*you*.

Only *you* can decide which food or drink to keep in your diet and eliminate those to which you are attached, feel a need to justify, or find yourself rationalizing, "This one time won't hurt." These items will continue to trip you up.

Also consider other diet-traps, such as baking things for others to show them love, or attending social events to seek someone's approval. Are these all potential saboteurs to your success? Can you demonstrate love or find approval in other ways?

Take time to study yourself, your needs, and your own behavior. This is the most important factor in your program.

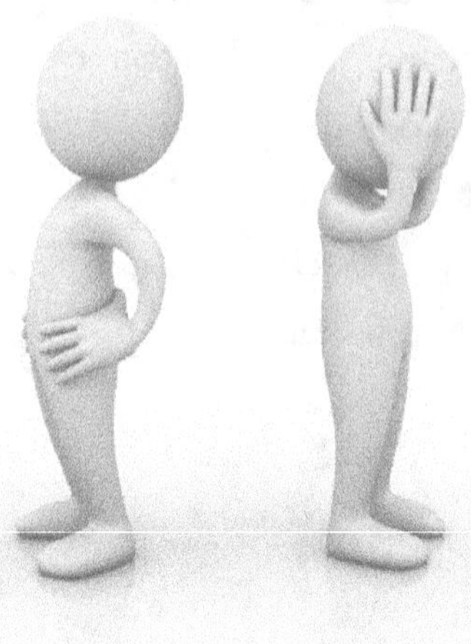

FORMULA BUSTER #19: CONFLICT IN RELATIONSHIPS

"Peace is not absence of conflict; it is the ability to handle conflict by peaceful means." —Ronald Reagan

Change can be fun. But watch out, because there are others in your life you must consider. To some extent, any alteration in your routine will impact those close to you. Nevertheless, you need to stay positive and unafraid. If the relationship is strong and loving, it will be flexible. It will survive and even thrive.

Some conflict is inevitable, but it need not paralyze you. Learn to work through each disagreement to develop tools that can help you now and in the future. If you can build up a toolbox of effective ways to resolve these skirmishes, you are well on your way to successful friendships, parenting, and a fantastic marriage.

Take a look at these three examples of problems that arose when people rearranged their personal boundaries.

CHAD'S STORY

Chad and his girlfriend were both overweight. They enjoyed a long-term relationship with each other and planned to marry.

He wanted to shape up, lose weight to feel better, and excel in his profession. The loss of weight would develop his confidence. He believed he deserved to live better, so he began the process of self-discovery. He set spiritual, financial, mental, and physical goals. These included a healthy diet and regular exercise.

As he began reaching those goals, he became more attractive and exuded great confidence. Because he was being true to himself, he reaped the rewards of his efforts. Soon after, his business took off.

His girlfriend became jealous of his success and felt threatened. She wasn't interested in losing weight or improving herself. Although Chad encouraged her to accompany him, she refused to join him. She even seemed to want to stay overweight and stagnant in her own personal life. They eventually called the wedding off and broke up.

Chad was upset that his ex-fiancée didn't want a better life for both of them, but he knew he was doing the right thing by moving on.

ROSEMARY'S STORY

Rosemary weighed 300 pounds, and food was her life. Although she said she wanted to lose weight, she never took action. Her excuse was she had been married for thirty-five years. She claimed a change in lifestyle would disrupt her marriage. She wasn't willing to risk doing something that would affect her relationship with her husband, even if it would be positive. To this day, she's still married and as heavy as ever.

BRICE'S STORY

Brice's buried emotions surfaced as overeating. He and his six siblings learned to avoid their alcoholic parents when they drank and became mean and angry. He grew up so consumed with sidestepping them he never got in touch with his own feelings.

In his twenties and with a degree in hand, he left home and began working full time. Even though he wasn't living at home anymore, negative feelings flooded his unconscious mind. He felt alone, isolated, and unable to develop lasting relationships.

During this time, he gave his life to Jesus. He knew the Christian life was the way for him, because he experienced great relief and security upon taking this step. Still, he felt something missing. He decided to find a Christian counselor, one who shared his spiritual beliefs, to talk about his troubling feelings.

To his surprise, his counselor suggested he held suppressed anger. This prevented him from honoring his feelings when relating to others—and himself. With the counselor's help, Brice realized his ways of communicating were flawed.

FORMULA FACTOR: COMMUNICATION

This is the information Brice followed to rid himself of anger. When conflict arose, he needed to identify where he was making mistakes in his communication with others. She explained the four outcomes of any conflict:

- I win; you lose.
- I lose; you win.
- I lose; you lose.
- I win; you win.

Now, if you look at the above list, which one do you think would contribute to a harmonious, long-term relationship? If you guessed "I win, you win," you're right.

If you're like me, though, you've probably fallen into one or more of the other categories at some point. I want to help you in the same way I've been helped, so I'll dig into each of these now.

I WIN; YOU LOSE.

This means I get my way 100% and you get your way 0%. This is an aggressive position taken by the winner, with lack of consideration to the loser's needs. The winner may not think they are being inconsiderate. They may think they are meeting their personal needs and establishing boundaries. They may want to be courageous and communicate what they say in the way they say it. What happens is they wind up distancing the other person at the expense of winning. For example, they could yell and intimidate the other person. They could be overly opinionated and drown out any opportunity for debate, or they could be closed to new ideas or input. In addition, over time the winner may have less respect for the loser who seems to be unwilling to speak up for himself.

I LOSE; YOU WIN.

This means I get my way 0% and you get your way 100%. This is a passive position taken by the loser. In this case, I'm being overly considerate of your needs and not meeting any of my own. The loser in this case may not hang around for long. For a marriage with two committed people, this could be an unhappy situation. The loser would probably become more distant and aloof over time, reluctant to share feelings or opinions for fear of being trampled upon. The marriage may stay intact, but it wouldn't be harmonious. Why would someone allow this to happen to themselves? Perhaps from a lack of courage.

You may not know the other person's past or what motivated them to behave in the way they do, but you do have a responsibility to act in a way that glorifies God and promotes peace in your relationships.

I LOSE; YOU LOSE.

This means there is no compromise and no one gets their way: a stalemate. Nothing for you and nothing for me in multiple ways. Neither party is considerate enough to meet either their own needs or that of the other. Neither is there courage to self-examine, to change oneself or the situation. This could, at worst, result in both people not speaking to the other indefinitely. At best, they find no resolution. No one will be happy.

I used to think people in this situation either didn't love each other or simply didn't care about the relationship. I've grown to believe that may be the case for some. For many, though, it may be a matter of lacking good communication tools or the willingness to grow personally.

I WIN; YOU WIN.

This doesn't mean you and I both get our ways 100%. What it does mean is we've reached a consensus where both members are reasonably satisfied with the outcome, in addition to maintaining honor for the other person. Do you get the difference here? It involves high consideration to yourself, to meet your personal needs, but also with a priority to respect the other person's needs. You must be assertive, yet rid yourself of pride, examine yourself to uncover any faults you may have, and put those aside for the sake of preserving and even edifying the relationship. In other words, the partnership is a greater priority than the individual.

Here is a summary of this information:

HIGH CONSIDERATION OF OTHERS

Passive/Low Courage	Assertive/High Courage
I LOSE/YOU WIN	I WIN/YOU WIN

LOW CONSIDERATION OF OTHERS

Passive/Low Courage	Aggressive/High Courage
I LOSE/YOU LOSE	I WIN/YOU LOSE

You may find your situation doesn't perfectly fit into these four categories. Yours may be a 50/50 split. What that should tell you is there's some work that needs to be done for one or the other party. This would greatly improve your relationship. The more you practice this, the better and more successful your experience will be.

You need to exercise compassion with your loved ones as you begin your road to change. You can accept them as they are and not expect or demand anything from them. You can take differences in stride, since you know you're doing what's right for yourself, yet others have the freedom to be themselves.

When you take this perspective, your partner may choose to join you. Others may opt to stay as they are. Regardless of their choices, you can have peace.

FORMULA BUSTER #20: STOWAWAY FOOD

"I can resist everything except temptation." —Oscar Wilde

We need to recognize another common problem. As long as there are others living with us, there will sometimes be food in the house we'd rather not have around.

Our goal isn't to have a cheat-proof home. However, these are some food challenges you may face:

- **The junk** your hubby, wife, partner, or roommate brought home today happens to be your favorite poison.

- **Your child** is such a picky eater you have stuff around the house you swore you would never buy or feed to him/her. This junk tempts you.

- **Leftovers** remain from the party or event you hosted, or some you were "coerced" into bringing home from the office party.

- **A lapse** in your own good judgment compelled you to buy something at the store you knew was bad for you.

FORMULA FACTOR: DON'T LOOK, DON'T TOUCH

I've had just as many successes as failures with this Formula Buster. Even though I know the tools, I know what I can do as an alternative, sometimes I simply don't feel like following my formula. Unfortunately, I pay the price afterwards: regret, remorse, and weight gain.

Am I being too hard on myself? Possibly. But why would I want to do something I know is going to hurt me? I want to wake up in the morning feeling great, not guilty. So is this a matter of self-discipline or adjusting my thinking so I don't feel poorly about myself?

I don't know what's right for you, but I can honestly say I shouldn't eat something if I'm not hungry or if my body doesn't need it. That should be enough for anyone to make a decision.

The question to these problems is, "What will you do about it?"

The right answer is, "Nothing!" *(As long as you don't eat it!)*

FORMULA BUSTER #21: S-S-STRESS

If you keep your mind free from the stress that causes you to eat, you will be less susceptible to indulge in tempting food at home. Your priority is to take care of your mind. Your biggest obstacle and challenge will be yourself—your willingness to protect yourself from overeating.

FORMULA FACTOR: PAUSE AND FOCUS

Do you know your own head games, the ones that sabotage your diet? When do you allow yourself to play them? These are dangerous luxuries. If you succumb too often, you'll have a hard time losing weight.

Keep focused on your goal, and you will be more likely to adhere to it. However, if you give in to temptation, don't beat on yourself later! Self-criticism may well set up another vicious cycle of stress that leads to more overeating.

FORMULA BUSTER #22: NO WATER QUOTA

"Water is the driving force of all nature." —Leonardo da Vinci

Do you remember the 8x8 rule for drinking water?[lxix] There is no scientific evidence that eight 8-ounce glasses of water per day (8x8) are the right amount of water for all healthy individuals.[lxx]

It is true that drinking too much water or not drinking enough can be harmful. For example, marathon runners who drink too much water without replacing electrolytes often wind up in the hospital getting intravenous fluids. Not drinking enough water can cause dehydration, which affects many bodily functions.

If we stay away from extremes, we will be fine.

FORMULA FACTOR: SET YOUR WATER QUOTA

The correct water quota is a daily amount you assess for yourself, based upon your lifestyle, health, climate, and medications. Stick loosely with this amount and modify it as needed. Other beverages and foods may also be included as part of the total water consumed.[lxxi]

The easiest way to tell if you are drinking enough water is to monitor the color of your urine: It should be clear or a very pale yellow in color, although some supplements and medications may also affect this. Measure a quantity of water to drink for one day and notice your urine's color. Then, follow the pattern your body sets for you. Let that be your guide.

The 8x8 rule does not take into account the water in the foods you eat, your size, activity level, or environment. So if you do use this rule, use it as a guideline only. If it works for you, this can be your daily quota.

You need additional water when you exercise or when it's hot outside. Every day will be different, so adjust your consumption accordingly.

Keep a glass at your desk and carry a refillable bottle in your car. Then plan to use the restroom more frequently!

FORMULA BUSTER #23: PEOPLE-PLEASING

"A friend to all is a friend to none." —Aristotle

Are you the type of person who says, "Yes" to someone's request before really checking out what that means to you?

If this is you, how many times have you regretted or even resented the fact you agreed to do something? After thinking, "Do I really want to do this?" Did you do it anyway, despite regret or resentment, because—after all—you committed to doing it? Do you think it would look bad to back out? Are you worried about what others may think if you did?

FORMULA FACTOR: PLEASE YOURSELF FIRST

Be true to yourself! Caring for other's needs before your own will sabotage your success with weight loss. If this is your natural tendency, you will need to change your response. You cannot be a people-pleaser if you want to succeed with your personal goals.

Focus on yourself first, even if you find this uncomfortable. Once you pay attention to your needs and communicate them to your friends or loved ones, you will be much happier. The best part is once you're in the habit of taking care of your needs first, then you are much more capable of helping others meet theirs.

If you are a people-pleaser, give yourself some time before accepting the next request. Say, "I'll get back with you." You will probably accept fewer opportunities, take better care of yourself…and be happier and thinner as a result.

FORMULA BUSTER #24: CRASH DIETING

"Self-discipline is often disguised as short-term pain, which often leads to long-term gains. The mistake many of us make is the need and want for short-term gains (immediate gratification), which often leads to long-term pain." —Charles F. Glassman

Advocates for fast weight loss believe a medically supervised crash diet is acceptable as a kick-start to a longer-term diet. The theory is quicker results will motivate and encourage the dieter to keep on the plan.

However, many liquid diets involve a radical restriction of calories. They may omit an entire food group and will confuse the metabolic process of the body. This can make it more difficult to lose weight unless the dieting is sustained. Furthermore, the dieter often puts socializing aside for a period to time in order to adhere to the strict program.

Unfortunately, most of the crash dieter's weight loss may be water. This will be regained when normal eating patterns resume. What was seen as a kick-start and a motivating factor winds up being a backlash and a discouragement. The victim might totally give up at this point, regaining more weight than he lost.

Have you ever gone on crash diets[lxxii] to lose your excess weight quickly for some event? Or have you simply found crash dieting an easier way to lose weight for a short period of time? This results in an all-or-nothing mentality. The truth is it is harder to eat moderately than not to eat at all! Have you ever wished God had made you without a need for food?

It is harder to eat moderately than not to eat at all!

FORMULA FACTOR: SLOW AND EASY WINS THE RACE

The key to losing weight is to develop habits that will enable you to maintain the weight. These take time to develop. They aren't impossible, but require persistence, determination, and support from others.

FORMULA BUSTER #25: HOLIDAY HOLDOVERS

"The consequences of today are determined by the actions of the past. To change your future, alter your decisions today." —Anonymous

There are several ways to approach the holidays:

- Ignore the fact there will be added temptations to eat fattening food and neglect to plan.

- Set unrealistic expectations for yourself.

- Approach these times realistically. Allow yourself more freedom than normal, while still staying within reasonable boundaries.

If you ignore the food challenge over the holidays, you are destined to find yourself with added weight at the beginning of the year. This is a discouraging place to be. You may feel overwhelmed and give up. You may not bother to set another New Year's resolution because you feel you will fail anyway. The extra pounds may stay on your body indefinitely.

On the other hand, an attempt to continue a strict diet regime over the holidays can be equally defeating. This swings the pendulum in the opposite direction. Your intentions are good, but they wind up causing more harm in the end.

Do you know yourself well enough to admit the holidays are super hard for you and food? This is the best place to start. From here, you can lower your expectations to overcome temptation. You can be easy on yourself and allow a bit more laxity with your formula. You can plan to exercise more frequently for the time, to compensate for the added calories.

FORMULA FACTOR: SPACE IT OUT

When you separate Thanksgiving and Christmas, you have four and a half weeks between the two days. There's another week before New Year's Eve. Keep these events separated in your mind, rather than taking the whole holiday season in one bite. It becomes more manageable.

Allow more time for meditation. Avoid the craziness. Do your shopping early in the day. Create white space in your calendar. Ask God to help you drive safely and defensively. Ask Him to help you moderate your food intake. Pray before eating. No, really—pray as if your life depended on it!

Create white space in your calendar.

Believe it or not, I get a kick out of watching all the crazies during the holiday season. I mean, people are insane! They don't realize how outside forces drive them to lose their serenity. It is so thrilling to be on the outside of this, looking in, especially since I used to be that way. You can have this empowerment too.

Magazines and advertisements stuff my mailbox. I don't even look at them. They go straight to the recycler. Instead of being bombarded with noise, I turn off the radio. I stay at home and shop online. I avoid the crowded, busy malls. I also spend within my means.

Strive at this time of year to maintain an emotional even keel. This is the first step to controlling your food. And remember, *you* are in control. No one or nothing can take your inner peace away from you unless you allow it.

SECTION III:
TOOLS FOR HEALTHY LIVING

"If it is to be, it is up to me." —William H. Johnsen

We've spoken about many principles of permanent weight loss. We'll briefly touch on many of the tools described in detail in the previous chapters and add a few more to our toolbox as well. These are in no particular order of importance, since that depends on you and your individual formula for healthy living.

Do you remember our talking about the diet never being static? Here are some examples:

- Nutritional needs change as you age.
- Metabolism slows as you age.
- Medical issues may come.
- You may develop sensitivity to certain foods.
- You may need more/fewer nutrients than before—certainly fewer calories!

Accordingly, you will need to amend your current tools as your life changes. Be proactive and develop resiliency. Don't be surprised when your life seems unstable for a while.

If you want permanent weight loss, you must adapt, not only with food, but also in how you relate to people and situations. As your life changes over time, eating behavior (on the outside) will more easily change as you grow emotionally and spiritually (on the inside). Improved eating habits become a by-product of your internal work. Subsequently, a synergy develops through your introspective efforts, and as you work on one aspect, the others get worked on simultaneously!

If this section is where you turned first when you picked up this book, you may be overwhelmed by all my suggestions. Try one or two for a few days. See how they work for you. Later, you can add or remove tools you want to keep or discard.

TOOL #1: WORK THE MOUTH, BUT NOT BY EATING

Can you find ways to socialize with others who share your interests? When you are busy with interesting, productive activities, you won't have the time or desire to overeat.

I often have an emotional craving to connect with someone, but if I'm not honest, I mistake that craving for hunger. It is easy to run to food for the solution instead of becoming still to get in touch with my real needs.

I also have tried substituting other things in my mouth for food. On my way home from France, I flew to Long Island to visit my mother for two weeks on my way to Houston. Once there, I experienced a similar isolation to that in Paris. The temptation to eat was strong, but here, I could see the red flag.

I accompanied my mom to the grocery store and purchased a multi-pack of gum for myself (about fifty sticks). I wanted to work my mouth, and I didn't want to eat. I thought the gum would help.

Well, I came home and proceeded to consume (yes, I ate) every stick of the gum. It didn't start out that way, of course. I only intended to chew some of it. But I learned an important lesson that day that I've never forgotten. *Don't try to substitute what I want to do (binge) by putting something else in my mouth.* Now, when in this situation, I go in the opposite direction. I read, call a friend, write in my journal, go for a walk, or clean house.

These are my suggestions: call a friend to talk on the phone, go to church early and mingle. Is there a small group you have a common interest with? Organize a weekly meeting to share ideas.

Remember the connection linking isolation, overeating, and depression. Take measures to prevent this downward spiral from occurring.

TOOL #2: FIND A PURPOSE

Haggai 1:5 was my Bible reading today. It motivated me to write and put everything else aside. Here's what I read:

Now this is what the Lord Almighty says: "Give careful thought to your ways. You have planted much, but harvested little. You eat, but never have enough. You drink, but never have your fill. You put on clothes, but are not warm. You earn wages, only to put them in a purse with holes in it." This is what the Lord Almighty says: "Give careful thought to your ways. Go up into the mountains and bring down timber and build the house, so that I may take pleasure in it and be honored," says the Lord.

I felt God's convicting hand upon me. I have so many urgent things to do, yet many of them don't advance goodness, truth, or God's kingdom. The reading was a call to assess my priorities and use the talents God gave me.

I am sure you have thoughts about activities you might want to try some time. There may be a book you want to write. You may also have a bucket list of things to do one day in the future. Well, I have news for you: *that day is here.* These are all indications of your heart's passions. God gave us the desires in our hearts. Our responsibility is to follow these dreams and work to make them reality.

HOMEWORK

In your journal, list three of these desires. Of those, choose one, and begin to let your creativity flow. Don't delay any longer. Before you know it, you may find yourself with incredible energy as you move toward your heart's goal.

TOOL #3: CALCULATE YOUR SUGAR GRAMS

I showed you in an earlier section about how to calculate the sugar grams in the foods you eat. But I can't emphasize enough how important this is, so I'm putting it as a tool here.

Visualization helps you understand how much sugar you're consuming. You can imagine cubes, restaurants packets, or actual teaspoons of sugar to help you see the quantity in a food item.

According to the American Heart Association (AHA), the maximum amount of added **sugars** you **should eat** in a day are:

- Men: 150 calories per day (37.5 grams or 9 teaspoons).

- Women: 100 calories per day (25 grams or 6 teaspoons).[lxxiii]

Here's the calculation:

$$\frac{\textbf{Number of Sugar Grams Per Serving}}{4} = \textbf{\# Teaspoons Sugar}$$

TOOL #4: MOVE IT—DAILY

By being active, you shift your focus from mental to physical. You do something positive and get the body involved, so you can't help but feel better.

On the lighter side of activity, go for a walk, weed the garden, do a load of laundry, organize a drawer, or tackle an overstuffed closet. This is an outward act to change your inward thinking and may or may not involve exercise. The point is to get your body moving toward something productive and your mind off eating.

Some ways to include this in your schedule are:

- Wake up a little earlier to do fifteen minutes of yoga.
- Take advantage of the fitness facility in your office building before work, during lunch, or after hours.
- Take a walk around the neighborhood each night after dinner.

When you become consistent with your schedule, exercise is so much easier. You won't have to think about it once it becomes a habit.

Moving your body is as much mental as it is physical. When you're aware of the connection between your mind and body, you will make fitness a priority.

TOOL #5: SWEAT

This one may take a while to accept. Some of you may never like it. But I guarantee you, once you are sold on sweating; you'll never go back to your old, indolent ways!

Plan to workout at least three times a week. Going on a hard bike ride, participating in an aerobics class, or doing an intense circuit for strength training does wonders for the soul. You will temporarily forget your worries because you're physically working hard. You'll purge impurities through your sweat glands. This is like taking a shower from the inside out.

TOOL #6: LEAVE THE KITCHEN

Physically remove yourself from temptation. Simply get out of the kitchen or leave the house if the craving is too great. Whatever you do, don't go back for at least thirty minutes.

Take a shower, brush your teeth, and involve yourself in something else.

If you are a follower of God, do you wonder why you still have temptations? God isn't the tempter, but He will allow you to be tested. This process will refine your faith if you make the right choices and turn toward God when you are agitated.

Remember this Scripture:

"No temptation has seized you except what is common to man. And God is faithful; he will not let you be tempted beyond what you can bear. But when you are tempted, he will also provide a way out so that you can stand up under it."— 1 Corinthians 10:13

TOOL #7: KNOW YOUR TRIGGERS

In Part 1, Section 13, we talked about the different types of triggers and how they can sabotage your efforts to lose weight and keep it off. If you're unclear about how they affect you, I encourage you to go back and re-read that portion.

Do you feel you *don't* have any triggers? If what I've written in this book has resonated with you, you may want to rethink the question.

If you think you may have triggers but don't know what they are, simply observe your eating behavior for the next week, then work the exercises from this section.

Your triggers are your friends. They alert you to deeper things going on within you and direct you toward healing. Don't be afraid of them, but instead trust them. They don't lie.

It takes courage to discover the things that cause you pain. It's so easy to avoid the real problem and head toward the food. This further hinders your growth, recovery, and permanent weight loss.

God has a beautiful plan for your life. He wants you to seek Him and to walk in His ways. Satan roars like a lion and causes fear, but he's harmless unless we take his bait. He wants you to destroy yourself, keep you away from truth, and prevent you from having an abundant life.

Don't let him do that to you!

TOOL #8: ELIMINATE MOST PROCESSED FOODS

There are so many additives in the foods we buy. The list seems to be getting longer and longer. Since most are unfamiliar, you may tend to ignore them, but that doesn't change the impact they have on your body. If I were to guess, I would say these additives are either unhealthy or nutritionally unnecessary.

What is a processed food, anyway? Anything produced with salt, additives, preservatives, refined flour, refined sugar, artificial flavor, fillers, emulsifiers, etc., etc… Even soy meats and soy cheeses are processed foods.

You don't have to be a chemist to know all about these things. It may be hard to completely eliminate all processed foods in your diet, too. Suffice it to say, the less you eat them, the healthier you will be.

TOOL #9: EAT MORE FOODS THAT RESEMBLE GOD'S CREATION

Instead of eating frozen broccoli with cheesy sauce, buy fresh broccoli and sprinkle some kind of real cheese on top. Yes, cheese is a processed food, but we will take this one step at a time! Rather than frosted cereal, switch to a healthier boxed version. Try some steel-cut oats for a change (they take a while to cook—soak them the night before so they soften quicker).

Check out the ingredients on muffins bought from the bakery. Then, find a simple, healthy recipe for homemade muffins and store them in the freezer.

These are just a few suggestions to help move you away from less healthy alternatives to better ones. The goal is to become aware of what you are putting in your body. Soon you will be able to make educated choices based upon your knowledge. You will have greater control over your diet and a healthier you.

TOOL #10: EAT MORE FREQUENTLY

This may seem a daunting task for those who eat one meal a day. Such frequent meals can also be a chore for those who are accustomed to a few meals a day.

The thought of eating so often is easier to stomach when you consider several of the meals are small snacks, not full meals. These mini-meals are portable and fast, so you don't have to stop what you're doing to eat them.

The goal regarding this frequency is not to increase metabolism, but to reach a place of satiety. The last thing you want when you're on a diet is to feel deprived. Eating frequent meals reduces this possibility.

You'll know what your ideal number of meals will be when you aren't mentally preoccupied with your eating. You also won't be famished prior to your next meal.

TOOL #11: ESTABLISH A WATER QUOTA

A water quota is the minimum amount you require yourself to drink most days to stay sufficiently hydrated. To establish a good quantity, consider your weight, the climate where you live, the season of the year, and your activity level. The key to knowing how much to drink is in the color of your urine: it should be light yellow. Some days you will need to drink more and others less. Setting a target for yourself will give you a baseline and keep you on a schedule.

Buy a quart-sized or liter-sized (approximately 32-ounce) refillable bottle. Carry it with you at all times. Bring it when you get in the car to run an errand. Choose water when you dine at a restaurant. You will be surprised at how easy your quota is to reach when you include water with the activities you already do.

However, don't go from one extreme to another. Increase your water intake gradually, and listen to your body—your ultimate guide.

TOOL #12: GET AS MUCH REST AS YOUR BODY NEEDS

When something is on your mind, do you have difficulty falling asleep? Perhaps a disagreement with your spouse is still unresolved. A crucial appointment the next day, a test, or a presentation can keep most of us awake.

If you never have a problem sleeping, you are blessed. For us lesser mortals, however, there is an ebb and flow. Some nights we sleep well, while others find us staring at the digital numbers of our bedside clock.

The lack of proper rest will break down our immune systems so we are more susceptible to illness. Rest—or the lack thereof—may well be related to our ability to lose weight.[lxxiv]

Some people use melatonin to help them sleep.[lxxv]

TOOL #13: CUT BACK OR ELIMINATE ALCOHOL

Alcohol is a definite obstacle to weight loss. To attempt to include alcohol with a diet will only frustrate you and slow down the process. Why? Excess, empty calories.

Alcohol	7 calories per gram
Protein	4 calories per gram
Fat	9 calories per gram
Carbohydrates	4 calories per gram[lxxvi]

Alcohol stimulates the appetite and causes you to eat more. It may also have a negative impact on your motivation to persevere with your program, particularly if you have reached a plateau.

If you find you have competing desires for drinking alcohol and losing weight, you might want to journal about this. Do you crave a drink when you are stressed out and use it as a tool to relax? Can you have one or two and then stop, or do you continue once you start? Most importantly, can you stop your alcohol consumption in order to reach your goal weight?

TOOL #14: CUT BACK OR ELIMINATE FAST FOOD

Have you ever heard these words or said them yourself? "I don't care what's in fast food. I just like the way it tastes."

Quality and good nutrition aren't usually found in fast food. You may be shocked at how these products are processed, along with all the artificial flavors and colors added to them. The more you learn about the substances you put into your body, the more nutritionally sound choices you will make. You will be healthier for life.

There is much evidence about the negative long-term impact too much fast food has on your health.

A very entertaining book about this topic is *Chew on This: Everything You Don't Want to Know About Fast Food* by Eric Schlosser and Charles Wilson. Also, an excellent documentary film you won't want to miss is "Super-Size Me," about a man who tried to subsist on McDonald's menu for a month. His weight ballooned; his energy plummeted; and he experienced terrifying side effects.

If you really love fast food, try to cut it back by one time each week. You will probably find that, in time, you will feel better and will lose the craving for it.

TOOL #15: MAKE A DECISION EACH DAY TO COMMIT TO YOUR PLAN, FOR TODAY ONLY

"I try to live my life one day at a time, and if I look too far in advance, I get really stressed." —Hope Solo

Wake up each day with determination to stick to your program for that one day. Have a plan and work it, taking one day at a time. Prepare your meals and carry them with you if necessary. Don't even think about what happened yesterday. Start each day fresh.

Consider whatever obstacles you might face that day, and expect to overcome them. If something didn't work for you before, try a different approach.

Let's say you are expected for a family dinner at an in-law's house tonight. They always serve high-calorie casseroles that give you indigestion. After the big meal some kind of sugary dessert will inevitably follow—your trigger food. You will be there at least four hours, listening to family stories about people and events you know nothing about. How can you plan for this event and yet stay in alignment with your goals?

You can do a number of things. Eating before you leave home will allow you to eat small portions, enough to taste and compliment the hostess. You might also take a small food item with you that you can eat discreetly. Always have a glass of water to take the edge off any nervousness. You can sip to your heart's content and stave off the jitters. You can also plan to excuse yourself to go for a short walk. Someone might even join you.

TOOL #16: PLAY WITH YOUR PET

"Until one has loved an animal, a part of one's soul remains unawakened."
—Anatole France

I love animals. My neighbor calls me Dr. Doolittle because I feed the stray cats, raccoons, possums, birds, and squirrels. My husband has seen me rescue birds, a possum, and even a bat. What would life be without these furry friends? Probably boring.

Pets are entertaining to watch and fun to own. Medical studies have proven they relieve stress and anxiety.[lxxvii] They definitely change our lifestyles, but they're worth the time and expense. Those who find the joys of pet ownership will always have them.

You can adopt a pet at your county animal shelter, the Humane Society, the SPCA, or other places. Pet supply stores also have regular adoption days.

TOOL #17: CUT OUT NON-FIBROUS CARBS AFTER 5 P.M.[lxxviii]

Non-fibrous carbohydrates are starchy carbohydrates, such as breads, pasta, chips, corn, legumes, potatoes, oatmeal, rice, and all forms of sugar. These carbs are the worst types to put into your body late in the day. You need them earlier to coincide with your energy needs. When eaten in the evening, they may wind up being stored as fat if you are not active enough.

Instead, have a double portion of veggies or a side salad in the evening. If still unsatisfied after your meal, make a cup of hot tea and wait at least thirty minutes before venturing back into the kitchen. You can also go to bed early.

If eating out, the restaurant's appetizer bread or chips may be an irresistible challenge. Go somewhere else or eat at home.

TOOL #18: PURCHASE MISCELLANEOUS MEASURING UTENSILS

Buy measuring spoons and cups of all sizes. Leave one in the oatmeal canister, nut jar, cereal box, or wherever you store your food. This trick will help you stay on track with portion control.

Do you feel like you're playing a juggling game? Portion control, the type of food, the time of day you eat it, emotional balance, and spiritual fulfillment—all play a part in weight control. Keep at it, and you'll get better as time goes on.

TOOL #19: PORTION YOUR FOOD IN ADVANCE

Designate one day a week to do all your cooking in advance. A good schedule might be when you return from the grocery store. This way, meat won't have to be frozen prior to cooking, and the end result will be a fresher, more satisfying meal.

Purchase five or six meal-sized food storage containers that will stack easily in the freezer. These should be large enough to hold a serving of protein, a veggie, and a starch. A good size would be about four inches wide by two inches tall. For soup, a pint-sized plastic container should be adequate for most people.

After you cook and cool your weekly meals, separate them into the storage containers directly from the baking dish or pot. You will now have a stockpile to grab from when on the run.

A small, one- to two-gallon insulated container is great for longer day trips to keep several meals fresh. This comes in handy if you spend a lot of time in the car.

Finally, if you purchase boxes of crackers, bags of nuts, or any other item of large quantity, pick up some plastic sandwich bags. When you're waiting for your food to cook (above), divvy single-sized portions into these bags. Doing so will remove the temptation to eat from the larger package. This will help you exercise portion control.

Proverbs 31 speaks about a wife of noble character. In verses 14-15, it reads, "She is like the merchant ships, bringing her food from afar. She gets up while it is still night; she provides food for her family and portions for her female servants."

One way we can model our lives after this person is to plan our meals and prepare them in advance.

TOOL #20: TAKE FOOD WITH YOU WHEREVER YOU GO

Have you ever suddenly found yourself starving with no alternative but a mini-mart or a fast food restaurant? *Prepare yourself daily to succeed!* This will take a little preplanning at first, but soon it will become such a way of life, you won't even think about it.

Experiment by taking different foods with you, such as pumpkin seeds, granola bars, cheese sticks, hard-boiled eggs, protein bars, protein drinks, veggies, or fruits. Store nonperishable emergency snacks in the glove compartment of the car. When you encounter the unexpected— being stuck in traffic, or a longer-than-expected meeting—you'll be prepared. Plus, if you have this food on hand, you won't arrive home famished. You will end the day strong and wake up the next morning victorious.

TOOL #21: USE THE SAME SIZED BOWL/PLATE

Once a food is measured into a correct serving, use the same sized plate or bowl. This technique is helpful to keep portions consistent. You may serve a bit more or less, but you know it will always be approximately the same.

Use this tool for cereal poured from its box or for entrees, like meats or chicken breasts. Your eyes will learn to gauge measurements, and you'll stay on track.

TOOL #22: H.A.L.T.

This is an acronym for "hungry, angry, lonely, or tired," four physical/emotional states that can throw anyone off balance. Never allow yourself to remain in any of these too long. Let's look at each of these.

Hungry—For someone who struggles with overeating and making right choices with food, this principle is critical to success. If you allow yourself to get too hungry, several things may occur. Your metabolism may take a dive, and your blood sugar may get low. You may get irritable and snappy at people. When the body gets out of whack, the mind becomes disordered—and vice versa. On the other hand, if you prepare meals in advance and keep food with you, you'll always have quick and healthy foods on hand. You will maintain steady blood sugar levels.

Angry—Many people struggle with anger and use it as an unhealthy tool to cope with life. Pay attention to your reactions. Do you automatically become angry in response to certain personalities or situations? As a child, anger may have served you well as a defense mechanism, but it's a definite detriment to adult relationships.

If you suffer from buried anger, you need to become aware of what makes you angry. How do you feel physically when this happens? What triggers it? Is there associated negative self-talk? This is an excellent time to pull out your journal. Write about your feelings as soon as you can when they arise. Otherwise, they may get buried again and prolong your recovery.

Some ways to rid yourself of anger are therapy, books, or workbooks with journaling exercises and questions. Remind yourself that you have made the decision to no longer carry this destructive emotion. Take constructive action. It's good to talk to a trusted friend who can listen and offer constructive advice. Above all, take your burdens to the Lord. Honest, repentant prayer will transform your life.

Lonely—Loneliness is preventable, but if you go too far without taking action, it can paralyze you. Once isolation reaches this point, you may become depressed.

Try to avoid this downward spiral. Look for signs you are drifting into loneliness. Are you isolating when you could be socializing? Are you cancelling activities you normally attend? Are you overeating more frequently? These could all be signs you are falling into an emotional state that may be difficult to recover from.

Stay involved in a fellowship or a club to prevent the onset. Work at developing friendships with people who will phone you when you are missed.

Tired—This one is a toughie. When I'm tired, everything seems off-balance. I tend to want to eat more when I'm tired, as if the extra food would give me more energy. That seems logical, but what my body is craving is rest, not food. Sometimes it is easier for me to put something in my mouth than lay my head down, but even a fifteen-minute catnap or meditation session can be beneficial.

TOOL #23: CHANGE YOUR MINDSET

"Your attitude, not your aptitude, will determine your altitude."
—Zig Ziglar

Your mindset is one of the few things you have complete control over. However, mastering the mind is never easy. Negative feelings pop into your head before you are aware of them. Once you've allowed this to happen, it is harder to dig yourself out of the pit.

Here's a reprinted work by Charles Swindoll:"[lxxix]

ATTITUDES

The longer I live, the more I realize the importance
of choosing the right attitude in life.
Attitude is more important than facts.
It is more important than your past;
more important than your education or financial situation;
more important than your circumstances, your successes, or your failures;
more important than what other people think, say or do.
It is more important than your appearance, your giftedness, or your skills.
It will make or break a company. It will cause a church to soar or sink.
It will make the difference between a happy home or a miserable home.
You have a choice each day regarding the attitude you will embrace.

Life is like a violin.
You can focus on the broken strings that dangle,
or you can play your life's melody on the one that remains.
You cannot change the years that have passed,
nor can you change the daily tick of the clock.
You cannot change the pace of your march toward your death.

You cannot change the decisions or the reactions of other people.
And you certainly cannot change the inevitable.
Those are the strings that dangle!
What you can do is play on the one string that remains—your attitude.
I am convinced that life is 10 percent what happens to me
and 90 percent how I react to it.
The same is true for you.

Chuck Swindoll

I have copied this and posted it in my office. I don't read it every day, but it gives inspiration when I need it. When I'm in a funk, reading this helps me pull myself up. I realize I have chosen to be unhappy and can choose a joyful perspective.

TOOL #24: TAKE A COURSE OR HIRE A PROFESSIONAL

If you have time and are inclined to further educate yourself in fitness or nutrition, you will benefit from the added knowledge. Sound information will help you make wiser choices. You will also associate with like-minded individuals who have similar goals. You may even make a new friend or ally who can help you stay focused. For those of you who want more extensive internal work, counseling may be an option. Make sure to choose a professional who can give you pure, objective, and educated feedback. Consider nutritionists, dieticians, personal trainers, life coaches, and others. Please don't hesitate if your conscience is guiding you in this direction. Working with a pro is a fantastic complement to your healthy life program.

TOOL #25: BE CONSCIOUS OF FATS IN YOUR DIET

Throughout this book, We've discussed fats quite a bit. Make it a habit to know how much fat is in everything you eat, so you won't even notice you're doing these calculations. The two things to remember are the fat calculation and the range of fat you want to stay within. Here's the formula:

$$\frac{\textbf{Calories From Fat Per Serving}}{\textbf{Total Calories Per Serving}} = \% \textbf{ Fat}$$

And the ideal range is to keep fat at 25-35% of your total daily calories.

If you're like me, you hate keeping track of things like this. It's just one more thing to think about. What I do is calculate the fat in what I purchase. I typically buy the same items over and over at the grocery store. But for new or unfamiliar items, I always do this calculation, keeping in mind my ideal range. Oftentimes, I'll return the item to the shelf. High-fat foods are simply not worth it to me anymore.

There's an inverse relationship between a high-fat food and the serving size. The higher fat, the smaller the serving should be. Almost always, I'll opt for the lower-fat/higher volume foods that satisfy me the most.

TOOL #26: PRACTICE SELF-EVALUATION

"Calm mind brings inner strength and self-confidence, so that's very important for good health." —Dalai Lama

If you become aware of something ripping you up inside, take a moment and stop whatever you're doing. Breathe deeply and clear your mind. Define the source of your stress. Is this something you have control over? Can you change it? Do you need to pray for guidance or direction? Or do you need to practice acceptance?

The simple act of a quick self-evaluation session can offer you a new perspective on what is upsetting you.

Take time to develop this habit. Persist until you have it down. You will be more relaxed and happy throughout your day and, ultimately, your life.

The benefit of taking these few moments of introspection will also provide you with new choices you may not have realized were available. Your life will be more productive and your relationships more harmonious.

TOOL #27: MAKE THE BETTER BAD CHOICE

I learned this principle from Keith Klein, a well-known and successful nutritionist in Houston, Texas. If you are tempted to eat something you know you shouldn't, try to bargain with yourself. For example, if you want cheesecake, think of another choice (decaf latte and biscotti, perhaps). This might satisfy you as well as the cheesecake.

This tool will allow you to have a "cheat" without too much damage to your eating plan. You can satisfy your craving without compromising your long-term goal of weight loss.

Often, cravings are spontaneous. When they occur, if you pause and make a better choice, the desire may go away.

TOOL #28: EAT AT RESTAURANTS LESS FREQUENTLY

"Achievement is largely the product of steadily raising one's levels of aspiration and expectation." —Jack Nicklaus

How often do you go to restaurants? Do you eat out for fun, as part of your profession, or both?

If you eat out for entertainment, you have total control over how often you go, but if you take clients to lunch or dinner as part of your profession, you may face more of a challenge. You may need to modify where you go, when you go, and what you eat. For example, instead of a dinner appointment, make it for lunch instead. If you must have an evening meeting, schedule it earlier rather than later. You will prevent weight gain if you have more time to burn calories after eating. The earlier you eat a high-calorie meal, the better.

If you eat out frequently, track your visits for one week or even a month. This will give you a starting point and help you determine what changes you need to make.

If you don't like to cook or if you enjoy the convenience of having someone else prepare your food, dining out can be a stumbling block for you. However, it may be necessary for you to cut down on restaurant eating—or eliminate it entirely for a while—in order to reach your goals.

Do you eat less healthfully at a restaurant? Is your caloric intake there more than with a meal at home? When dining out, do you eat foods not kept in your pantry? If you answered yes to any of these questions, it may be easier to lose weight to cook at home more and eat out less.

If restaurant food is a temptation to you, two options are:

- **Remove it**. If you are tempted by endless bowls or plates of chips, crackers, or bread, you may ask the waiter not to bring them to your table. At home, if portion control of a particular food is a problem, simply don't buy or bring it home.

- **Remove yourself from it**. After removing the temptation, you may still be enticed by certain menu items not on your program. If you order those, you will find yourself eating in a way that is not honorable to yourself. Perhaps the best option is to avoid going to that particular restaurant altogether, or at least decrease the frequency of your visits.

Before you go to a restaurant, call a friend who has similar struggles and understands your predicament. Tell them what you plan to eat. This builds accountability and can motivate you to stay on track.

Truthfulness will determine your success. Why are you going to a certain restaurant? Is it because you really want to give in to your craving? Be honest with yourself. On the other hand, is there another restaurant where you will be less tempted? Or do you not feel like striving toward your goal today?

Your choices are yours, but the consequences of your choices are also yours.

TOOL #29: LOOK AT THE MENU BEFORE YOU ARRIVE AT THE RESTAURANT

"The commander must decide how he will fight the battle before it begins. He must then decide who he will use the military effort at his disposal to force the battle to swing the way he wishes it to go; he must make the enemy dance to his tune from the beginning and not vice versa." —Viscount Montgomery of Alamein

Before leaving home and when you're not hungry, look at the restaurant's online menu and decide what you will order. Look for lean, low-calorie, or low-fat options. You will choose best by making your decision in advance.

Right before you leave, eat a small snack—a glass of skim milk, a cheese stick, or a piece of fruit. You'll have more willpower to make the best decisions.

Suppose your friend wants to meet at a restaurant that tempts you with its fare. You might cave and order things you'll later regret. Share your goals with your friend and ask for her support.

The time for successful planning is before you are surrounded by the ambiance, so you arrive at the restaurant with strength and determination to succeed.

TOOL #30: LOOK FORWARD TO SOMETHING EACH DAY

"I get up every morning determined to both change the world and to have one hell of a good time. Sometimes, this makes planning the day difficult."
—E. B. White

One day, I was down in the dumps and talking to a friend about everything I didn't like about life. She asked me a question and gave me some advice that completely changed my viewpoint. "What are you looking forward to today?" and "List twenty things you are grateful for right now."

I had to stop and think about it, but as I wrote, I realized I had much to anticipate each day and for which to feel grateful. Among the things I listed were my morning meditation, a hot cup of perfect coffee, and the joy of petting my cats.

I can choose today what I focus on. When I see positive things in my life, I have a good day. On the contrary, if I look for the negative, my day can quickly turn sour.

TOOL #31: SET GOALS BEFORE YOU RETIRE AT NIGHT

Before you retire at night, make a short list of things you would like to accomplish the next day. When you wake up the next morning, you'll have a sense of purpose and direction. You'll also have determination to accomplish these goals, which will increase your motivation.

Structure your time around these tasks and you'll have a more productive day. If you do this every day, you will accomplish so much more in life.

TOOL #32: CHECK YOUR HORMONE LEVELS

Do you have mood swings that effect your eating? Do you feel your hormones (or lack of them) are somewhat to blame? You can anticipate these swings by charting them. If you find a consistent pattern each month, you might have a hormonal imbalance. You may benefit from a doctor's advice. Hormone replacement therapy is a personal decision. If you suspect you might have this problem, ask your OB-GYN to schedule blood tests. You may experience both physical and emotional relief as a result.

TOOL #33: PRAY & MEDITATE

"You can do more than pray after you have prayed; but you can never do more than pray until you have prayed." —A. J. Gordon
"We live, in fact, in a world starved for solitude, silence, and privacy, and therefore starved for meditation and true friendship." —C. S. Lewis

Prayer was mentioned earlier as something to do when you wake up in the morning, but prayer can be an effective tool during the day as well.

Whenever you feel stressed, frustrated, upset, or out of control, stop and say a prayer. A simple prayer can work wonders. Try something like, "God, I don't know what is going on with me, but I feel all messed up and twisted inside. I know that when I feel this way, I want to do nothing but eat. I know that eating will not solve my problem. Please help me to see my problem clearly so that I don't have to hurt myself by overeating today. Amen."

Finally, allow a few minutes of quiet time each morning to connect with God. This regular meeting is the most important part of your day. It can help you deal with any unexpected circumstance that might happen, because you established your unity with Him in the morning.

Meditation is an amazing way to relax our bodies and minds and put them in sync, so we can make the best choices. Select an inspiring verse and reflect on it over and over. One of mine is,

"Finally, brothers, whatever is true, whatever is noble, whatever is right, whatever is pure, whatever is lovely, whatever is admirable—if anything is excellent or praiseworthy—think about such things." —Philippians 4:8

It took me a long time before I was a true advocate for this method of calming my mind. If you have never meditated, stay open to the idea, and try it. It's worth every minute you invest in the endeavor.

TOOL #34: READ NUTRITION LABELS

Establish the habit of reading nutrition labels every time you grocery shop. This one routine will help you be aware of what you're consuming, compare to other like products, choose wisely, and take control over your health.

In an earlier section, I asked you to set some ideals regarding your diet. For example, keep fat grams 25-35% of total calories, opt for low-sodium versions of foods, or try to eliminate sugars in most foods. Reading labels will help you attain these goals. You will be successful in your weight loss efforts because you'll be armed with the facts.

TOOL #35: INCORPORATE JUICING[lxxx] IN YOUR REGIMEN

For years, I thought people who juiced were extremists. I didn't want to do anything extreme, so I stayed away from it.

Later, my husband and I watched several documentaries on juicing and health. We were totally amazed at the ideas presented and went out to buy a juicer. We started it as a means to add nutrition to our diets, and we have continued it since.

One of my unhealthy patterns is I tend to be all-or-nothing with certain behaviors. The way I acted in the past is, "If it's good, then more will be better!" I saw the danger of overdoing, so we've never done a juice fast. Part of my recovery from unhealthy food habits involves getting away from these extreme behaviors. I may do a juice fast one day, but not yet. Meanwhile, I'll do regular juicing.

I am sure there are fantastic benefits to juice fasting. Information abounds on the subject. But for you, if extremism is an issue, stay away from it unless it is medically supervised.

Juicing floods your bloodstream with super-nutrients that can only come from fresh fruits and vegetables. Because the juice is liquid and doesn't require much digestion, it enters your bloodstream even quicker. Most juicing vegetables have a low glycemic index too.

One more note on juicing: when I began, I started with fruits only. They tasted good, but I quickly realized the amount of fructose entering my body was too high. Because I am sensitive to high amounts of any type of sugar in my system, I changed from fruits to vegetables only. I continue this today. If I want a fruit, I eat the whole fruit so my body must work harder to break it down. This also maintains the roughage often lost in the juicing process.

TOOL #36: SUBSTITUTE APPLESAUCE FOR OIL IN BAKED SWEET GOODS

Try substituting no-sugar-added applesauce in oil-based baked goods, such as quick breads, muffins, and some cakes. You will notice a slight change in taste and texture (typically sweeter and softer), but you'll save your body hundreds of fat calories.

Most sources recommend a one-to-one swap of oil or fat to applesauce, e.g., if the recipe calls for one cup of oil, substitute with one cup of applesauce.

If you'd rather ease your way into this substitution, use half applesauce and half oil. If satisfied with the finished product, next time slightly increase the ratio of applesauce to oil. You may be able to do without oil completely, or you might find as little as one or two tablespoons of oil added to the applesauce is ideal.

TOOL #37: KNOW THAT YOU ARE IN CONTROL

Do you eat what you crave, or do you crave what you eat? Think about it. If you have a craving, it may be a superficial desire for sugar, flour, or some other kind of comfort food, or your body may be alerting you that you are nutritionally deficient in something. It is possible your body has lost its ability to comprehend what it needs. Instead, it craves what your mind decides it wants.

You now know you are the master over your body because you have learned how to reset your metabolism through specific actions. You have the power to adjust your eating so you crave only the things you truly need, while treating yourself periodically.

Change your diet gradually in order to reap lasting results. Be patient with yourself. One fine day, you will find you no longer want what you used to crave, and what you want to eat is what your body really needs.

Try this once and see how you feel: when you have a craving for junk, drink a cup of vegetable juice. I guarantee you will feel great with no desire to eat empty calories.

TOOL #38: MAKE A CUP OF HOT TEA OR COFFEE

Whether a ritual, a comfort, a relaxing activity, or a social custom, sipping a cup of hot tea or coffee can be soothing to our souls.

When craving something you shouldn't eat, try making yourself a cup of tea instead. Drink it away from the kitchen and focus on relaxation. This will make all the difference in your state of mind.

TOOL #39: PLAN YOUR FOOD "VACATIONS"

When you go on a vacation, you don't spontaneously get up and leave town that day. Plans must be made, arrangements set up, pet caregivers called, and lists noted of things to bring. You have to consider the rest of the family, their schedules, work schedules, cancellations, and events. The planning could be one day, a month, or even a year ahead of the actual event. Anticipation of that special day makes you look forward to it even more.

You do the same thing when you plan to indulge on a "food vacation." A date next Saturday with your significant other can be even more special when you take time to select which restaurant to go to and what to wear. A weeklong vacation could be a longer food vacation, but will require more preparation.

Balance is the key. What better way to motivate yourselves than to get thoroughly disgusted with your eating habits when you're on vacation? When you get home, you'll be so ready to get back on track. So relax and enjoy! Just remember there will be consequences to overindulging. Keep this in mind so you will "indulge in moderation." Does that sound like an oxymoron?

So the point of a food vacation is to take a break from the focus of the diet. It's a respite from the monotony and routine. Your intent will be never to stray too far from your good habits you've worked so hard to establish. You will always look forward to getting back on track.

If you keep these ideas in your mind when you plan your event, you will do so wisely. You will take certain foods with you and leave others at home. You will keep up with your water quota and avoid dehydration. You will carry snacks with you so you don't find yourself hungry without something healthy to eat. You will maintain control over your formula.

TOOL #40: CONTROL YOUR BLOOD SUGAR

Create a fat-burning environment in your body by choosing the right combination of foods. Don't allow your blood sugar to get too high (you overeat or indulge in sugary foods) or too low (by not eating frequently enough). Both overeating and/or under-eating will cloud your thinking, and you won't function well.

Be proactive, and plan your meals in advance. Utilize the glycemic index as a guide.

TOOL #41: KEEP YOURSELF MOTIVATED

If you move too slowly toward your goals, you might not recognize much benefit of your program. This can undermine your motivation and discourage you. On the other hand, if you persevere and are determined to reach your goals, you will more likely see noticeable results. You will be excited and energized to press on.

So how do you self-motivate? It starts with your desire to have the healthy body you seek. Keep your long-term goals in the forefront of your mind, and it will become easier to sacrifice short-term satisfaction.

Some great ways to inspire yourself can be found by watching any sport. It's impressive to watch an athlete perform with such ease, when in reality, what they do is difficult. Watching the young people compete in the Olympics is also a great way to cultivate desire for a healthy, strong body. You can always watch replays of these on YouTube.

Another way to get excited about your goals is to look in magazines with pictures of beautiful bodies or on-line clothing catalogs with models. These images will help you visualize where you want to be. Even though their size may not be realistic for you, the emotions stirred while viewing them will get you going in the right direction.

Don't forget about the cruise, vacation, wedding, or family reunion next summer. These events can be just the thing to stir you to action. There is a set timeline between now and then, and you can plan your work accordingly.

Be accountable to someone on a daily or weekly basis, for this little discipline will keep you on your toes. Talk to a friend periodically about your goals. If you really want to be motivated, you will find a way.

TOOL #42: POST QUOTES AROUND YOUR WORKSPACE

Inspirational quotes are a great way to make your environment more positive. Post them on your mirror so you see them as you prepare for your day. Tape them to the perimeter of your computer. Place them inside your wallet. Memorize quotes you can recite in your head as you wait in traffic or in the grocery store.

Here are a few inspirational quotes I have around my space:

- "A quitter never wins, and a winner never quits." —Vince Lombardi, Napoleon Hill, Proverb
- "God put me here to be happy; not being happy is my choice." —Unknown Author
- "You have to give before you can get." —Robert Collier
- "If you cannot do great things, do small things in a great way." —Napoleon Hill
- "The virtue of contentment destroys ungratefulness, restlessness, and dissatisfaction." —Unknown Author

Can you think of quotes or sayings that inspire you? List them in the front of your journal. Create an inspirational and uplifting workspace at your desk.

TOOL #43: APPLY THE 6-P RULE TO YOUR LIFE

"By failing to prepare you are preparing to fail." —Benjamin Franklin

The 6-P-Rule stands for, "Proper planning prevents pitifully poor performance." Remember this idea when you consider your day. You will be more likely to adhere to your goals.

Thoughts lead to actions,

Actions lead to habits,

Habits become your character, and

Character determines your destiny.

The hardest part of the program is the planning phase. Hopefully, you've been establishing your formula since the beginning of the book. You know now it will be different for everyone. Once you have chosen yours, you may occasionally face obstacles. However, your basic plan will keep you on track.

Remember, life is all about modification. You'll never stop

modifying!

Self-sabotage is a cunning thing. A little decision (or lack of decision) can place obstacles in your own path. You may say you want to change your life, yet it is easy to fall into self-defeating patterns—procrastination, comfort eating, etc.

Do you fail to plan? Can you identify areas where you have set yourself up for failure? If you can identify them, you can overcome them. You will start to realize the results you truly want.

TOOL #44: BELIEVE IN YOURSELF

Find a support group or network to help you achieve your desires. It doesn't have to be a meeting or an organization, only a handful of like-minded friends. The point is to surround yourself with people who will affirm your character, build you up, and help you recognize your potential. You are God's masterpiece, designed for a unique purpose. Supporting friends will help you become all you are meant to be.

If you are faced with a difficult situation at home or the office, the group will help you stand strong. Stay close to your encouragers, and rely on their strength, not yours.

You are worthy of achieving weight loss. You are capable of doing so. Believe in yourself. When you wake up each day, make the decision to follow your program toward radiant health. Keep your self-talk positive at all times.

TOOL #45: MAKE IT SIMPLE

Simple is best for eighty percent of your meals. Make it easy on yourself to eat a clean and lean diet. Make your grocery list and shop every week. Prepare your meals in advance. Stock your fridge with a variety of pre-cooked meals you can heat and eat. Make this as routine as brushing your teeth. In fact, this process can even be a little boring at times. But then again, so is brushing your teeth!

TOOL #46: DON'T ROW IN THAT RIVER

A good friend of mine said to me once, "Don't row in that river." The "river" could be hanging around a person who is a bad influence on you, being around tempting food that wears your defenses down, or behaving in ways that are harmful to you or to others.

Become proactive and observe your thoughts. For example, if you have a relationship with someone who mocks your efforts to change your lifestyle, do whatever you can to avoid that person. If you are around tempting food, either remove yourself or the food. If your thoughts are negative, be aware of them and repeat a positive affirmation instead.

If you don't want to row in that river, take steps to become free from the situation. Decide you want real freedom, and do what is needed to achieve it.

If you find yourself succumbing to negative temptations, recognize your responsibility to change your thinking patterns. If you allow yourself to continue this behavior, it will become a habit and your self-esteem will crash as you realize you have not been true to yourself.

TOOL #47: WRITE IT OUT, DON'T STUFF IT DOWN

The first thing every morning when you wake, take a few moments to journal. During your day, write about the feelings that threaten to overwhelm you. Learn the art of jotting your thoughts down on paper to help you become adept at processing your feelings. With practice, you'll get better. You will become quick to identify troubling thoughts that used to drive you to the kitchen. You will acquire tools to effectively counter these thoughts and be able to refrain from overeating. You will lose weight and keep it off.

Instead of turning to food to stuff unwanted feelings down, honor yourself by acknowledging your feelings. Those unwanted cravings will eventually go away.

TOOL #48: THEIR URGENCY IS NOT MY EMERGENCY

I wish someone had told me earlier in my life that when someone around me is stirring up drama, I am not required to participate, but I missed that information and wound up causing myself unnecessary problems that I could have avoided.

Now that I know this, I no longer have to be a part of anyone's chaos. They can have it all to themselves. I'm a happier, more peaceful person as a result of letting others own all of their mess. Stay away from crazy people!

TOOL #49: GO ON A ROMANTIC DATE

You take the initiative here and ask your spouse (or romantic partner) out. Schedule it on the calendar, and plan what you will do. Anticipate the evening, spending quality time with your favorite person. Look your best to feel and behave that way too. Enjoy!

TOOL #50: SIT OUTSIDE AND BREATHE IN NATURE

As long as the mosquitoes aren't bad and the temperature is moderate, this is worth making time for. Leave your cell phone inside the house for twenty minutes. How often do you simply sit outside and notice God's miracle in your backyard? You can look at it as a form of meditation. You will gain perspective, allowing your mind to wander. It won't take long for you to realize how fortunate you truly are.

CONCLUSION

As you become closer to your goal, you may find losing the last few pounds much harder than the first. What you need to do is hone your program even further and apply more of these tools simultaneously. If you do, you will continue to get results.

I will close with a poem called, "It Couldn't Be Done,"[lxxxi] by Edgar A. Guest:

Somebody said that it couldn't be done,
But he, with a chuckle, replied
That "Maybe it couldn't," but he would be one
Who wouldn't say so till he'd tried.
So he buckled right in with the trace of a grin
On his face. If he worried, he hid it.
He started to sing as he tackled the thing
That couldn't be done, and he did it!
Somebody scoffed, "Oh, you'll never do that;
At least no one ever has done it;"
But he took off his coat and he took off his hat
And the first thing we knew he'd begun it.
With a lift of his chin and a bit of a grin,

Without any doubting or quiddit,
He started to sing as he tackled the thing
That couldn't be done, and he did it.
There are thousands to tell you it cannot be done,
There are thousands to prophesy failure,
There are thousands to point out to you one by one,
The dangers that wait to assail you.
But just buckle in with a bit of a grin,
Just take off your coat and go to it;
Just start in to sing as you tackle the thing
That "cannot be done," and you'll do it.

Remember: It's not any one thing you do, but rather a lot of little things you do, that will produce the results you want!

ABOUT THE AUTHOR

Annette Radvansky has been a personal trainer since 1994, and recently began writing. This first book was borne from a desire to share everything she knew about weight loss, first from her personal experience and then from what she learned as she trained individuals with similar struggles. She currently resides in The Woodlands, Texas with her husband and daughter. Find out more or contact Annette at www.annetteradvansky.com.

BIBLIOGRAPHY

i.   John Wooden & Steve Jamison, *Wooden: A Lifetime of Observations & Reflections*. New York City: McGraw-Hill, 1997.

ii.   Now called "The Steps to Freedom in Christ."

iii.   Neil T. Anderson, *The Bondage Breaker*. Harvest House Publishers. Eugene, Oregon, 1990.

iv.   Life Application Study, NIV, Character description of Thomas, Paragraph 4, p.1927.

v.   From *Fifteen Questions*. Copyright 2012 by Overeaters Anonymous, Inc. Reprinted by permission of Overeaters Anonymous, Inc.

vi.   https://en.wikipedia.org/wiki/Willy_Wonka_%26_the_Chocolate_Factory

vii.   http://www.prevention.com/food/healthy-eating-tips/the-57-names-of-sugar

viii.   https://www.ncbi.nlm.nih.gov/pubmed/19943985
https://www.nsca.com/education/articles/ptq/meal_frequency_and_weight_loss
https://www.instantknockout.com/ik/can-meal-frequency-affect-weight-loss/

ix.   https://www.health.harvard.edu/diet-and-weight-loss/eating-frequency-and-weight-loss

x.   https://www.sciencedaily.com/releases/2017/07/170720094844.htm

xi.   https://www.webmd.com/diet/a-z/3-hour-diet

xii.   http://www.webmd.com/food-recipes/features/how-food-affects-your-moods#1

xiii.   www.fda.gov/Food/DietarySupplements/

xiv.   https://www.amazon.com/Nature-Valley-Crunchy-Granola-Honey/dp/B008BLFCK8

xv.   https://www.google.com/search?q=kellogg's+pop+tarts+frosted+brown+sugar+cinnamon+nutrition+image&client=safari&rls=en&tbm=isch&source=iu&pf=m&ictx=1&fir=i9Y2HFa-bN2GqM%3A%2Cx9yifXpuH3YBuM%2C_&usg=__8Wv208qM_DxZ6N2hqhTCIl0boNE=&sa=X&ved=0ahUKEwi87PDj1InXAhUISiYKHeZWBHcQ9QEINTAA#imgrc=bLRgUgAqrnqjtM:

xvi.   http://www.myfitnesspal.com/food/calories/kirkland-costco-einstein-bros-plain-bagel-407619442

xvii.   https://www.hy-vee.com/grocery/PD5650300/Sara-Lee-Deluxe-Bagels-Plain-6-CT

xviii.   http://www.fatsecret.com/calories-nutrition/usda/coconut-milk-or-cream-(liquid-canned)?portionid=35347&portionamount=0.250

xix.   http://www.myfitnesspal.com/food/calories/dairyland-1-cup-2-milk-180252943

xx.   http://panogoldpics.com/vh-breads.html

xxi.   http://www.zingbasket.com/food-for-life-ezekiel-4-9-sprouted-grain-bread-flax.html

xxii.   https://www.livestrong.com/article/314019-the-side-effects-of-calcium-propionate/
https://en.wikipedia.org/wiki/Calcium_propanoate

xxiii. Production of bread using sodium stearoyl lactylate as a replacement for shortening Original Research Article
Food Research International, Volume 25, Issue 4, 1992, Pages 285-288
Basil S. Kamel, R. Hoover

xxiv. http://www.myfitnesspal.com/food/calories/heb-bulk-in-shell-snow-white-pumpkin-seeds-474733916

xxv. https://mobile.fatsecret.com/calories-nutrition/planters/cinnamon-pecans

xxvi. https://www.fatsecret.com/calories-nutrition/generic/chicken-breast-skinless

xxvii. https://www.fooducate.com/app#!page=product&id=421D213E-A004-11E1-882E-1231381BE564

xxviii. https://www.fooducate.com/app#!page=product&id=55B6D586-C414-D76C-4C4F-A7AAD5391EAE

xxix. https://www.jennieo.com/products/3-extra-lean-ground-turkey-breast

xxx. A Guide To Federal Food Labeling Requirements For Meat, Poultry and Egg Products, P. 85-86, 91, 96
U.S. Food and Drug Administration
10903 New Hampshire Avenue
Silver Spring, MD 20993
1-888-INFO-FDA (1-888-463-6332)

xxxi. http://www.myfitnesspal.com/food/calories/broccoli-raw-425578799

xxxii. https://www.greengiant.com/products/detail/green-giant-steamers-broccoli-cheese-sauce-10-oz-box/

xxxiii. https://www.google.com/search?client=safari&rls=en&q=white+rice+nutrition+facts&ie=UTF-8&oe=UTF-8

xxxiv. https://www.google.com/search?client=safari&rls=en&q=cooked+wild+rice+nutrition+facts&oq=cooked+wild+rice+nutrition+facts&gs_l=psy-ab.3...236303.237338.0.237582.7.6.0.0.0.0.0..0.0....0...1.1.64.psy-ab..7.0.0....0.DOHz2nssCBI

xxxv. https://www.google.com/search?client=safari&rls=en&q=brown+rice+nutrition+facts&ie=UTF-8&oe=UTF-8

xxxvi. https://www.google.com/search?client=safari&rls=en&q=half+and+half+nutrition+facts&oq=half+and+half+nutrition+facts&gs_l=psy-ab.3...86634.88489.0.88861.13.8.0.0.0.0.0..0.0....0...1.1.64.psy-ab..13.0.0....0.kKMMGn-KVL4

xxxvii. https://www.target.com/p/nestle-174-coffee-mate-original-coffee-creamer-35-3oz/-/A-14056736

xxxviii. https://www.medicalnewstoday.com/articles/141442.php

xxxix. Natural Statins: How to lower cholesterol levels.
www.newportnaturalhealth.com

xl. British Heart Foundation: High cholesterol. NHS Choices: High cholesterol – Prevention. The New England Journal of Medicine, Vol. 347, No. 19, Nov. 7, 2002;

xli. https://www.cdc.gov/cholesterol/facts.htm

xlii. https://www.fooducate.com/app#!page=product&id=DFCE515E-DEF3-11E1-956E-1231381BA074

xliii. https://www.amazon.com/Betty-Crocker-Chocolate-Muffin-Pouch/dp/B000EMQG16

xliv. http://www.myfitnesspal.com/food/calories/548498829

xlv.   http://www.myfitnesspal.com/food/calories/442896700

xlvi.   https://www.amazon.com/LABRADA-NUTRITION-Convenient-Go-Replacement/dp/B00166BBXW/ref=sr_1_7_s_it?s=hpc&ie=UTF8&qid=1509052154&sr=1-7&keywords=ready+to+drink+protein+shakes&th=1

xlvii.   https://www.amazon.com/Labrada-Protein-Non-GMO-Natural-Ingredients/dp/B06VYD73KJ/ref=sr_1_2_s_it?s=hpc&ie=UTF8&qid=1509052471&sr=1-2&keywords=protein+bar+labrada

xlviii. Meal Replacements: Choose Those Bars and Drinks Carefully Or How to Successfully Eat on the Run
By Kathleen M. Zelman, MPH, RD, LD
WebMD Weight Loss Clinic - Expert Column

xlix.   https://www.google.com/search?q=land+o+lakes+butter+nutrition+label+image&client=safari&rls=en&tbm=isch&source=iu&pf=m&ictx=1&fir=ULKc5rXBoCrYvM%3A%2CcHWPHtktUdZ2kM%2C_&usg=__n54OJ1MyXDpDJqrlOIbH2mHr1ic=&sa=X&ved=0ahUKEwjC1caS2frWAhUHXRoKHXZiA-EQ9QEIQDAL#imgrc=ULKc5rXBoCrYvM:

l.   https://www.google.com/search?q=pam+non+stick+spray+nutrition+label+image&client=safari&rls=en&tbm=isch&source=iu&pf=m&ictx=1&fir=e6YUeVcCPVgEhM%3A%2CGbhcZun78jJfFM%2C_&usg=__KBmZ0PSpeWH-TkWBASsXNkKvO9M=&sa=X&ved=0ahUKEwjNzN--2frWAhULnBoKHVV9DsYQ9QEINTAA#imgrc=e6YUeVcCPVgEhM:

li.   https://www.google.com/search?client=safari&rls=en&q=whole+egg+nutrition+info&ie=UTF-8&oe=UTF-8

lii.   https://www.google.com/search?client=safari&rls=en&q=egg+white+nutrition+info&ie=UTF-8&oe=UTF-8

liii.   https://www.google.com/search?client=safari&rls=en&tbm=isch&sa=1&q=strawberry+yogurt+nutrition+label&oq=strawberry+yogurt+nutrition+label&gs_l=psy-ab.3..0j0i7i30k1l2.75740.75740.0.78470.1.1.0.0.0.0.186.186.0j1.1.0....0...1.1.64.psy-ab..0.1.186....0.5sDWDhw1spk#imgrc=h6uaMqOXyBR3GM:

liv.   http://www.calorieking.com/foods/calories-in-yogurts-plain-fat-free-yogurt_f-ZmlkPTYxMzg5.html

lv.   https://www.google.com/search?client=safari&rls=en&q=raisins+nutrition+facts&ie=UTF-8&oe=UTF-8

lvi.   https://www.google.com/search?client=safari&rls=en&q=banana+nutrition+facts&ie=UTF-8&oe=UTF-8

lvii.   https://en.wikipedia.org/wiki/High-fructose_corn_syrup

lviii.   http://www.minneapolismn.gov/www/groups/public/@health/documents/webcontent/convert_264742.pdf

lix.   Hull, C. L. (1935). The Conflicting Psychologies of Learning: A Way Out. Psychological Review, 42, 491-516.

lx.   American Heart Association Guidelines. (n.d.). *www.heart.org*. Retrieved February 19, 2012, from http://www.heart.org/HEARTORG/GettingHealthy/PhysicalActivity/StartWalking/American-Heart-Association-Guidelines_UCM_307976_Article.jsp#.TzwpTHbCMYY
The effect of exercise on depression, anxiety and other mood states: a review

lxi.   A Byrne, DG Byrne - Journal of psychosomatic research, 1993 – Elsevier 46. JR Hughes; Psychological effects of habitual aerobic exercise: A critical review. Prevent Med, lxii. 13 (1984), pp. 66–78. ... 47. AD Simons, MS McGowan, LH Epstein, DJ Kupfer; Exercise as a treatment for depression: An update. Clin Psychol Rev, 5 (1985), pp. 553–568. ...

lxiii. 1 Authoritynutrition.com/9-fixes-for-weight-hormones/
2 healthline.com/health/diabetes/insulin-and-glucagon#overview1

lxiv. "Glycemic Index Defined". Glycemic Research Institute. Copyright 2006-2010, www.glycemicindex.com

lxv. Taken from chart on http://www.glycemicedge.com/glycemic-index-chart/

lxvi. http://www.dummies.com/food-drink/special-diets/glycemic-index-diet/defining-low-medium-and-high-glycemic-foods/

lxvii. Understandingthebibleway.com/sermon-outlines.html
Contentment: The Virtue And Value Of Contentment.

lxviii. "Do not conform any longer to the pattern of this world, but be transformed by the renewing of your mind" (Romans 12:2 NIV).

lxix. http://kandieshealthandfitnessproject.blogspot.com/2012/11/khfp-week-one-8x8-rule-of-drinking-water.html

lxx. https://geiselmed.dartmouth.edu/news/publications/news_digest/digest0802/myth.shtml

lxxi. http://www.webmd.com/parenting/features/healthy-beverages

lxxii. http://straighthealth.com/pages/articles/darticles/crash-diets-dont-work.html

lxxiii. https://www.healthline.com/nutrition/how-much-sugar-per-day

lxxiv. "Sleep More, Weigh Less," http://www.webmd.com/diet/sleep-and-weightloss

lxxv. "Melatonin and Sleep," https://sleepfoundation.org/sleep-topics/melatonin-and-sleep

lxxvi. http://nutristrategy.com/nutrition/calories.htm

lxxvii. http://science.howstuffworks.com/life/pets-happiness1.htm

lxxviii. http://discovergoodnutrition.com/2012/09/13/carb-cutoff-at-night/

lxxix. Copyright © 1981, 1982, by Charles R. Swindoll, Inc. All rights reserved worldwide. Used by permission. www.insight.org.

lxxx. Calbom, C., Keane, M., <u>Juicing for Life: A Guide to the Benefits of Fresh Fruit and Vegetable Juicing 1991.</u>

lxxxi. Public domain https://www.poets.org/poetsorg/poem/it-couldnt-be-done

ADDITIONAL READING

1. Campbell, T., Campbell T.M. II, The China Study, 2006.
2. Kravitz, Len et al., "A Review of the Impact of Exercise on Cholesterol Levels."
3. Rolfes S.R, Whitney E. Understanding Nutrition, 3rd edition, 2005.
4. Duyff, Roberta Larson, *American Dietetic Association Complete Food and Nutrition Guide* (revised and updated 3rd ed.) 2006.
5. Lee, H.H.C., Gerrior, S.A., Smith, J.A., "Energy, macronutrient, and food intakes in relation to energy compensation in consumers who drink different types of milk". *The American Journal of Clinical Nutrition* 66 (4): 616–23, 1998.
6. http://www.forbes.com/sites/alicegwalton/2013/09/04/the-6-weight-loss-tips-that-science-actually-knows-work
7. Puetz, T. *Psychological Bulletin*, November 2006. News release, University of Georgia.
   Better Sleep Found by Exercising on a Regular Basis.
8. Breus, M. J., *Exercise improves sleep, but it takes time to reap the benefits.* September 6, 2013.
9. White, J.R., Case, D. A., McWhirter, D., Mattison, A. M., *Enhanced sexual behavior in exercising men.*
10. Tuormaa, T. E., *The adverse effects of food additives on health: a review of the literature with a special emphasis on childhood hyperactivity,* Journal of Orthomolecular Medicine, 1994 - orthomolecular.org
11. Zinczenko, D., Goulding, M., Rodale, Eat This, Not That! 2013: The No-Diet Weight Loss Solution, 2013.
12. Steward, H. L., Bethea, M., Andrews, S., Balart, L. A., The New Sugar Busters! Cut Sugar to Trim Fat, 2003.
13. Dufty, W., Sugar Blues, Reissue edition, 1986.
14. Peeke, Pamela, Fight Fat After Forty: The Revolutionary Three-Pronged Approach That Will Break Your Stress-Fat Cycle and Make You Healthy, Fit, and Trim for Life, 2001.
15. Wolf, Ronni , Wolf, Danny, Rudikoff, Donald, Parish, L. C., *Nutrition and water: drinking eight glasses of water a day ensures proper skin hydration—myth or reality?*